Happy Birthday
May 1980
Love, Annies

How to Beat a Bad Back

HOW TO BEAT A BAD BACK

Hundreds of things to do to achieve a pain-free back

Including exciting new techniques to relieve back pain fast—plus a 13-minute-a-day medically approved exercise program for a life-long better back

Shirley Linde

Foreword by C. Norman Shealy, M.D., Ph.D.

Rawson, Wade Publishers, Inc. • New York

Library of Congress Cataloging in Publication Data

Linde, Shirley Motter.
    How to beat a bad back.

    Includes index.
    1. Backache.   2. Exercise therapy.   I. Title.
RD768.L62 1979   617'.5   79-64202
ISBN 0-89256-105-X
ISBN 0-89256-113-0 pbk.

Published simultaneously in Canada by McClelland and Stewart, Ltd.
Composition by Connecticut Printers, Inc., Hartford, Connecticut
Printed and bound by R. R. Donnelley & Sons, Crawfordsville, Indiana
Designed by Gene Siegel
Illustrated by Robert P. Kelley

To Scott and Bob

Acknowledgments

I wish to thank the following individual physicians, researchers, and organizations that make up some of the people whose work is quoted in this book or who have helped provide material incorporated into it.

Acupuncture Treatment Groups, New York; American Academy of Family Physicians; American Academy of Pediatrics; American Association of Retired Persons; American College of Sports Medicine; American College of Surgeons; American Medical Association; American Osteopathic Association; American Rheumatism Association; Dr. Gordon W. D. Armstrong, University of Ottawa, Canada; Arthritis Foundation; Prof. Ana Aslan, Institutul National de Gerontologie Si Geriatrie, Bucharest, Romania; Ruth Ann Aust, Honolulu; Dr. Louis V. Avioli, Washington University School of Medicine.

Bio-Medical Data; Blue Cross/Blue Shield; Dr. Steven F. Brena, Emory University Pain Control Center; Dr. C. Harmon Brown and Dr. Jack Wilmore, American College of Sports Medicine; Dr. Mark D. Brown and Dr. Robert Daroff, Spine Research Center of University of Miami School of Medicine, Florida; Al Buehler, Duke University, Center for Medical Consumers and Health Care Information; Dr. Norman F. Childers, Rutgers University; Dr. Theodore Cole, University of Minnesota; Dr. William F. Collins, Yale Medical School; Dr. Thomas Coyle, Bridgeport, Connecticut; Crozer-Chester Medical Center, Chester, Pennsylvania.

Dr. Eugene Dabezies and Dr. Michael Brunet, Louisiana State University; Dr. Ross Davis, Veterans Administration Hospital, Miami, Florida; Dr. Kenneth DeHaven, Cleveland Clinic, Department of Health, Education, and Welfare; Diagnostic Data; Dr. Ronald Dougherty, Syracuse, New York; Dr. Barbara Drinkwater, University of California Institute of Environmental Stress; Duke University; Dr. George E. Ehrlich, Temple University School of Medicine, Philadelphia; *Emergency Medicine*, Dr. Robert England, Philadelphia College of Osteopathic Medicine; Everest and Jennings.

Dr. Henry L. Feffer, George Washington University; Dr. Roger J. Ferguson, University of Pittsburgh; Dr. William Finney and Dr. D. Graham Slaughter, Baltimore; Dr. James Garrick, director of the St. Francis Center for Sports Medicine in San Francisco, and Dr. Ralph Requa, research director for the Margaret Goldwater Foundation for Research and Education, Sun City, Arizona; Göteborg University, Göteborg, Sweden; Dr. James Greenwood, Jr., Baylor University College of Medicine; Dr. John A. I. Grossman, George Washington University Medical Center, Washington, D.C.; Dr. Anders Hakelius, Karolinska Institut, Copenhagen; George Hickok, Diagnostic Data; Dr. Thomas Holmes, Dr. Richard Rahe, and Dr. Theodore Dorpat, University of Washington, Seattle; Dr. Ronald L. Huston, University of Cincinnati.

Internist News; Institute of Experimental and Clinical Medicine, Lithuania; Institutul National de Gerontologie Si Geriatrie, Bucharest, Romania; Dr. Douglas Jackson, University of California at Irvine; Dr. Monroe Jacobs, President, Podiatry Association of New York; John Hopkins University; Dr. Robert E. Kappler, Chicago College of Osteopathic Medicine; Dr. Jennifer Kelsey, Yale University; Micki King, U.S. Air Force Academy; Dr. Hans Kraus, New York University; Dr. Harvey Kravitz, American Academy of Pediatrics; Dr. Richard Kroening and Dr. David Bresler, University of California at Los Angeles.

Dr. Myron M. LaBan, Dr. Richard Burk, and Dr. Ernest Johnson, Ohio State University; Dr. Ronald M. Lawrence, American Medical Joggers Association; Dr. Charles LeRoy Lowman, Orthopedic Hospital, Los Angeles; Dr. C. H. Li, Hormone Research Laboratory, San Francisco; Lufthansa; Dr. John Marshall, The Hospital for Special Surgery, New York; Dr. John H.

McMaster, University of Pittsburgh; Mead Johnson Company; *Medical World News;* Dr. John M. Mennel, Veterans Administration Hospital, Martinez, California; Menninger Foundation; Merck, Sharp and Dohme; Dr. Arthur Michele, New York Medical College; Dr. John J. Miller, Miller Pharmaceutical Company; Dr. Milton Mintz, St. Clare's Hospital, Denville, New Jersey; Dr. Jerome H. Modell, University of Florida College of Medicine; Dr. C. G. Moertel, Mayo Clinic; Dr. Marilyn Moffat, New York University; Dr. Vert Mooney, University of Texas Southwestern Medical School.

Dr. Alf Nachemson and Dr. Gosta Elfstrom, Sweden; Dr. Willibald Nagler, New York Hospital–Cornell Medical Center; National Institute of Drug Abuse; New York Hospital–Cornell Medical Center; New York University Medical Center Institute of Rehabilitation Medicine; Dr. James A. Nicholas, New York Jets; Dr. Eugene S. Nordby, University of Wisconsin School of Medicine; Dr. George Northup, American Osteopathic Association; Dr. Burton Onofrio, Mayo Clinic; Dr. J. Blair Pace, Rancho Los Amigos Hospital, Downey, California; Dr. Gideon Panter, New York Hospital–Cornell Medical Center; Dr. Jack J. Pinsky, City of Hope Pain Center; President's Council on Physical Fitness and Sports.

Dr. James H. Renwick, London School of Hygiene and Tropical Medicine; Riker Laboratories; Roche Laboratories; Dr. Eugene Rogers and Dr. Barry Vilkin, Chicago Medical School; Dr. Hubert L. Rosomoff, University of Miami School of Medicine, Florida; Dr. John Sarno, Institute of Rehabilitation Medicine, New York; Dr. Christopher D. Saudek, Cornell University Medical College; Dr. Keith Sehnert, Center for Continuing Education, Georgetown University; Dr. C. Norman Shealy, Pain and Health Rehabilitation Center, La Crosse, Wisconsin; Dr. Peter Simkin, University of Washington; Simmons Company; Dr. Bernard H. Singsen, University of Southern California; Smith, Kline and French; Dr. Lyman Smith, Northwestern University; Dr. Clive C. Solomons, University of Colorado Medical Center; Jacki Sorensen, Aerobic Dancing Studio, Northridge, California; *Sports Medicine;* Steelcase; Dr. Richard A. Sternbach, director of Pain Treatment Center at Scripps Clinic in La Jolla, California; Dr. Richard M. Suinn, Colorado State University; Dr. Alfred B. Swanson, Blodgett Memorial Hospital, Grand Rapids, Michigan.

Dr. T. V. Taylor, University Hospital of South Manchester, England; Dr. Joseph S. Torg, University of Pennsylvania School of Medicine, Philadelphia, Pennsylvania; Dr. Jack de la Torre, University of Chicago; Dr. Joan Ullyot, Institute of Health Research, San Francisco; U.S. Food and Drug Administration; U.S. Department of Agriculture; United States Olympic Committee; U.S. Senate Committee on Nutrition and Human Needs; University of California; University of Iowa; University of Miami School of Medicine Spine Research Center; University of Texas Health Science Center, San Antonio.

Dr. Morton Walker, Stamford, Connecticut; Dr. Lionel A. Walpin, Cedars-Sinai Medical Center, Los Angeles; Dr. Sonja Weber, Columbia-Presbyterian Hospital, New York; Dr. Louise Wensel, Acupuncture Institute and Research Center, Washington, D.C.; Dr. Nils Westlin and Dr. Bo Nilsson, General Hospital, Malmo, Sweden; Dr. Jay A. Wiersma, Blodgett Memorial Hospital, Grand Rapids, Michigan; Dr. Leon Wiltse and Dr. Patrick Rocchio, Long Beach, California; Dr. Harold Wolff, Cornell University; YWCA of U.S.A.

Special thanks is given to Robert P. Kelley, of the Chicago College of Osteopathic Medicine, who provided the bulk of the illustrations used in *How to Beat a Bad Back*. The drawings in chapters three and six are courtesy of Dr. Arthur Michele, author of *Orthotherapy* (M. Evans Publishing Company, New York, N.Y.).

Foreword

by C. Norman Shealy, M.D., Ph.D.*

This is a book which ideally will receive the kind of public recognition that it deserves. If every American were to read and heed the outstanding collection of information and recommendations offered in this book, we might stem the tide of the 400,000 laminectomies performed annually. In my opinion, of the laminectomies that have been performed over the past twenty years, not more than 10 percent, at most, were indicated.

As far as osteoarthritis is concerned, virtually every human being at some point in life will have *X-ray* evidence of what is diagnosed as osteoarthritis. In most people the condition causes no pain, so don't be misled by a physician who tells you that you have osteoarthritis which will get progressively worse, as one of my patients was told. That patient is now working full time and is free of pain, three years later.

In general people who are physically active, reasonably well adjusted to their social situation, and who eat a well-balanced diet rarely have back pain of any significance. If you do have back pain the treatment of choice is likely to be acupuncture, or transcutaneous electrical nerve stimulation, or gentle spinal mobilization. In more extreme cases gravity reduction traction is the treatment of choice. All of these techniques are outlined in this

* Founder and Senior Dolorologist, Pain and Health Rehabilitation Center, La Crosse, Wisconsin. President, American Holistic Medical Association.

book. Probably in not more than one percent of patients with fairly severe back pain is surgery ever indicated. When surgery is recommended, unless you have true paralysis of the foot (foot drop), seek a second opinion. If the second opinion also suggests the need for surgery, seek a third opinion. If the third physician recommends surgery, then it is likely that you need surgery. If one of the three does not feel surgery is indicated, then you are better off following a conservative program.

In general, people with back pain have weak abdominal muscles and poor posture. *How to Beat a Bad Back* emphasizes ways to overcome both of these. It also shows you how to reprogram bad back habits in a positive rather than negative way for a better and stronger back. It shows you how to sit straight, reach for objects in a way that protects your back, hold the phone in such a way that your neck can maintain its normal position, maintain your ideal weight and stand tall.

In relation to the neck, I certainly agree with the comments in this book: sleep on your side or back; maintain a neutral posture of the head and neck both sitting and walking; shift your position frequently while sitting; sit in areas that are free of drafts or blowing air conditioning; sleep in a reclining posture; if you read while lying down, be certain that your head is in a normal neutral position; stand straight; maintain a normal ideal weight.

My personal preference in a mattress is a good foam rubber one (not polyurethane foam but real foam rubber) with about 32 pounds per square inch compressibility. We have found this to be the single most effective mattress for people with a wide variety of back problems. The so-called orthopedic and chiropractic mattresses are very firm and in my opinion often cause back pain rather than ease it. In general, people should avoid using pillows. If a pillow is necessary, the softest down pillow possible should be used.

In relation to osteoporosis, I do not believe that estrogen should be given. Women who remain physically active and take good doses of vitamin E are not likely to need such an artificial and potentially harmful substance.

Before I reproduce this book itself, I suggest that you read on. Follow the excellent advice and exercise programs herein and enjoy increased energy and the happiness of improved health.

Table of Contents

How to Beat a Bad Back

1 Why This Book Was Written

   . . . Because almost everyone has a back problem at one time or another.

   . . . Because, except for general checkups, *back problems are now reported to be the number one complaint of patients going to the doctor.*

   . . . Because doctors are reporting an astounding increase in the frequency and severity of back problems in both children and adults of all ages. More and more people are affected every year, until today back problems have reached epidemic proportions, touching every segment of the population.

   . . . Because much of the back pain we suffer is unnecessary and can be prevented or cured. People need not have the pain that they do.

   . . . Because having a strong back can make you better at work, at sex, at sports, as well as feel and look better.

   . . . Because the current literature presents only one point of view. This is the first time that information from all the experts has been gathered in one place.

Back pain has plagued mankind for thousands of years. Descriptions of back pain are found in the writings of Hippocrates and in the Bible. One anthropological theory is that cavemen and women were stooped over because they had arthritis and other back problems from living in damp caves.

Most of us take our backs for granted, assuming that they are there and will continue to function without trouble throughout life. But we can no longer assume this. The chances are good that most of us, even if we have a back that seems normal now, may suffer pain and disability in the future.

.It may happen gradually with everyday stresses and strains, diet deficiencies, tension, and lack of exercise gradually causing nagging pains and eventually serious trouble. Or it may happen suddenly with no warning. You may be shoveling snow, or bending over to raise a stuck window, or simply reaching down to pick up a toothbrush from the floor . . . when a stab of pain rips through your back, and you may not be able to straighten up. It can hurt and cripple you for the rest of your life. Some of us have had it happen already.

The statistics on the pervasiveness of back pain are astounding.

It is estimated that on any given day, *6.5 million people* are in bed because of back pain.

Doctors say four out of every five people in the United States can now expect to experience back trouble at some time in their lives! New cases are reported to appear at the rate of about 1.5 million per month. One health expert estimates there will be about *two billion* back patients in the next decade and one million practitioners treating them.

Victims have ranged from John and Edward Kennedy to Wilbur Mills and Elizabeth Taylor and the woman next door.

At many back pain clinics there is a five- to six-month waiting list to get an appointment because so many people need help. Thirteen states now claim low back pain as the leading cause of hospitalization.

Doctors say it is our most expensive disease, and the expenses to the patient can be truly astronomical. One thirty-two-year-old woman reported expenses of $160,000 over eight years. One doctor said a patient came to him having spent $450,000 out of his, or his insurance company's, pocket. The emotional cost of pain in terms of unhappiness and crippled lives is even higher.

And the cost to society is high in lost wages and productivity and in compensation payments. In the state of Washington, one out of four days lost from work is due to back disorders. In Massachusetts, the number one cause of claims on disability income policies is back problems. In Wisconsin, insurance experts say 75 percent of compensation payments go to back patients, who represent only 3 percent of compensation patients. In California last year, insurance companies paid out some $200 million to back patients. Even the most conservative estimates say that every year the nation loses 200 million workdays as a result of back disorders.

The problem is not limited to the United States. In Sweden, back-related conditions account for the greatest number of premature retirement and disability claims. In England, the government has decided to establish a chain of back treatment centers throughout the country because back problems are responsible for so much invalidism and absenteeism.

Back problems have become so common that many people simply have accepted living with their pain and misery, accepting it stoically as almost a natural part of their lives. They often don't even think of going to a doctor for help, and when they do go, in many instances they do not get adequate help; instead, despite the fact that there are many things that can help an ailing back, patients are often simply told to learn to live with their pain. Or they are subjected to surgery that they really don't need.

Indeed, one back specialist told a group of doctors at a scientific meeting that throughout the country "thousands of back sufferers are being misdiagnosed, improperly treated, and given little or no advice on proper back care."

But things *can* be done. The spine is not just an anatomical hat rack on which to hang the body's muscles and organs. The back is not a permanent fixture that cannot be helped if it is damaged.

There *is* help for the ailing back. A strong back can be made stronger, and a weak back can be made better. Even persons with severe problems, who are about to undergo surgery, can sometimes help their backs by doing exercises before surgery, can exercise to help restore strength afterward, or many times can even exercise to *avoid surgery.*

There are techniques to tone the muscles, improve posture, stretch ligaments, relax nerves, increase flexibility, reduce pain, and increase function.

How to Beat a Bad Back is written to bring these techniques to you. There is no other book that brings to the reader such widespread and detailed information from around the world on how to have a better back, including some research so new it has not yet made its way from the research labs to the office of the practicing physician, let alone the patient.

How to Beat a Bad Back describes all the different kinds of back troubles and tells what to do for them. It tells you why often-ignored stomach and buttocks muscles are vital to protect your back. It tells who is likely to get a bad back; if you are in a profession dangerous to your back; why strong people, even former athletes, may still be likely to have back trouble. It gives you tests so you can check yourself and your family for potential trouble. It tells you about lifting, and posture, and diet, and how to drive a car to best avoid backache, and the best ways to sleep, and how to work to give your back the most protection. It tells the periods in every man and woman's life when they are most likely to suffer back trouble. And it tells you how life-style and tension can affect your back, and what you can do about them.

The book's entire approach can be summed up in that fine, popular new word "holistic"—it looks at the entire person and all phases of life that affect the back, and it combines expertise and advice not just from one viewpoint but from *all* professions—the AMA, osteopaths, Olympic coaches, and others—bringing together for the first time knowledge and help integrated from all these groups.

Whether you have a bad back and want to make it better, or have a good back and want to make it even stronger so you can be better in sports, sex, and everyday activities and prevent future problems, this book is for you.

Doctors say that people cause 90 percent of their own back troubles because unknowingly they are doing the wrong things to their backs. *How to Beat a Bad Back* tells you the *right* things to do. It tells you the most important steps to take right now to reduce the likelihood that back trouble will ever strike you, for it is almost inevitable that as you age, you *will* have back trouble unless you take definite steps now to prevent it. And if you already have trouble, it will tell you what to do to get your back strong again and prevent future trouble, because if you have trouble once, even mild trouble, then the chances are strong you will have worse trouble in the future. Today's twinge can be tomorrow's excruciating pain that cripples your back and your life. That first back pain can be your back's signal for help. Unless you do something now, you can expect a bigger problem ahead.

The Better Back Program gives you conditioning exercises and other advice gathered from back experts around the world and puts them together into one program, the only one of its kind. By following the program, you can strengthen key muscles, stretch tight areas, and restore normal function. By knowing the necessary techniques, you can be your own training coach—your own therapist—to improve your back. It's easy, takes only a few minutes a day, mostly flat on your back. And the program works. Even if your back hurts you every day, the exclusive exercise program can make it possible for you to once more have a *good* back so that you can swim with vigor, walk without pain, and feel good again.

2 The Better Back Quiz

Most of us don't even think about our backs unless they start to give us trouble. Most of us know almost nothing about back problems until we develop a particular one ourselves.

How much do you know? Test yourself with this quiz. The answers may very much surprise you.

1. How many people currently have back trouble?
   (a) 100,000; (b) 1 million; (c) 10 million; (d) 75 million.
2. Bad backs are the most frequent reason for people coming to the doctor's office.   True or false?
3. What are the chances of your becoming the victim of a bad back?
   (a) 1 in 1000; (b) 1 in 100; (c) 1 in 10; (d) 1 in 4.
4. The number of bad back sufferers is increasing in alarming proportions. True or false?
5. Who is most likely to get back trouble?
   (a) a ditch digger; (b) a desk worker; (c) a runner; (d) a person who does not engage in sports or exercise.
6. Which groups have a lot of back problems?
   (a) men; (b) women; (c) blacks; (d) whites.
7. Children almost never have back problems. True or false?
8. The wrong kind of exercises, even common ones, can aggravate a back problem. True or false?
9. How you drive your car, the chairs you sit on, the mattresses

you choose, even expensive ones, can aggravate a back problem. True or false?

10. Which of the following are frequent causes of back problems? (a) muscle strain; (b) heredity; (c) kidney disease; (d) an ulcer; (e) prostate problems; (f) emotional tension.

11. Back trouble will always show up as some kind of pain in the back. True or false?

12. If you only have occasional back problems and they go away, it's okay to ignore them. True or false?

Answers

1. (d) 75 million people in the United States suffer from various types of back pain, according to the Arthritis Foundation. Bad backs are the number one claim on disability insurance policies. In fact, health insurance companies report about 28 million victims hobble and hunch their way to doctors for treatment each year. Many others have pain and stiffness and lack of mobility but haven't yet gone to seek professional help.

2. True. When the government did a recent survey of 235 million office visits to family doctors, the most frequent reason for the visit was shown to be a general physical checkup; but when patients went to the doctor's office with a specific complaint, by far the biggest complaint was a back problem, leading all other causes, even sore throats, colds, and stomach aches. A bad back is also the second most frequent cause of absenteeism from work. (Colds and flu are number one.)

3. (d) 1 in 4, most doctors say; although some back experts say it's closer to 1 in 3, and one doctor claimed 80 percent of all people will have back pain to some extent in their lives.

4. True. Nearly every physician I interviewed reported a great increase in the number of people coming to the office with back complaints. National surveys show the same increase on a general basis throughout the nation.

5. (b) and (d) Sedentary people.

6. (a) (b) (c) (d) All are correct. Every sex, race, and social group today has back problems, although some seem to be bothered more than others.

7. False. Even children have back problems. They can have posture problems, crooked spines, and other early-occurring back

conditions. Doctors are reporting a high incidence of disk problems in teen-agers, often even in 11- and 12-year-olds. Every age is vulnerable to back trouble.

8. True. Even simple exercises like bending down and touching your toes can cause back damage in some people. Doctors report that many patients come to them with problems caused by improper exercises and warn that even some of the exercises given to schoolchildren are dangerous.

9. True. Many are too soft, or do not give support in proper places. There are specific guidelines that can be followed to help counteract the situation.

10. (a) (b) (c) (d) (e) and (f). All of these conditions and many others can cause back problems. Many people believe that all bad backs are caused by pulled muscles or slipped disks, but there are many other causes. Only by checking them all out can you know for sure what is really causing your problem.

11. False. You may have back trouble and never have had a back pain in your life. The pain may show up later, or it may appear as pains in the ankles, thighs, or calves, never giving you a hint of where the trouble really originates.

12. False. An occasional pain now may mean a lot of pain later. It's always best to check out medical problems early so they can be corrected by simple, inexpensive means before they get serious. Best of all, follow the recommended procedures to give you a strong healthy back so that you will never have the problems that plague so many others.

More details are given about all of these and other questions later in the book.

3 At-Home Back Tests You Can Do Yourself

These are the tests done by physicians when they examine their patients for back problems. These tests do not take the place of a regular physical checkup, but there is no reason why you cannot run through them at home from time to time between your regular medical checkups to test both adults and children in your family for any abnormalities or weaknesses that could mean trouble in the future. If you find any symptoms or signs of a problem, or anything that is questionable, see your doctor and tell him what you found.

SIX DANGER SIGNS THAT COULD MEAN TROUBLE

Run your fingers carefully down the spine and see if you feel any extra-deep dimples, indentations, or blank spaces between the vertebrae.

Run your fingers down again slowly and feel for any small masses or strange extra bumps.

Check both sides of the spinal column for areas of increased oil or sweat production.

In a three-way mirror look along the spine for hairy patches or groups of hairs in a tuft like a small brush. They often indicate abnormalities in the spine underneath.

Press all along the spine, along the pelvic bones, and over the lower back on each side to see if there is any tenderness.

Check for mobility by standing straight, then bending to the right and to the left, then twisting to the right and to the left. Are you mobile, or stiff with limited motion? Is there pain?

Sit on the floor absolutely upright and straight (*not* leaning backward) and with the legs fully extended straight ahead. You should be able to keep your legs fully extended and flat to the floor without pain or difficulty and without falling backward.

You can check yourself for these signs or observe while others in your family do these tests. If there are any of these signs, it can indicate an abnormality in the spine or a condition that could cause serious future problems. Call your doctor to discuss further investigation.

CHECKING FOR LORDOSIS

It is normal for the back to have a slight curve, but too much of a curving arch is called lordosis and puts a strain on the back that can lead to trouble.

Stand sideways and observe your posture in a full-length mirror, or have the person you are checking in your family stand sideways in front of you.

Compare the curve in your back with the figures.

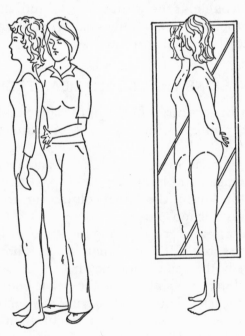

CHECKING FOR PELVIC TILT

Stand up straight in front of the person who is checking you. Have them observe the following on you. (It may help to level a yardstick across your body.)

Are the shoulders even or is one higher than the other?

Are the shoulder blades even and symmetrical?

Is one earlobe closer to the shoulder on one side than the other?

Is the spine straight, or does it curve to one side?

Look at the buttocks and hips. Are the two sides symmetrical, or are the creases different on one side?

Is one hip higher than the other?

You can also check for pelvic tilt by putting ink markings on each of the vertebra, being careful to keep the overlying skin in its normal position. See if the markings make a straight path, or whether the spine curves.

Doctors also frequently check for pelvic tilt by tying a weight to a length of string about two feet long and holding the end of the string against the bony vertebra that sticks out most at the bottom of the neck. The weight should fall exactly in the midline, following the spine and falling evenly in the midline of the crease between the buttocks. If the weight falls to either side, it indicates a tilt to one side of the back or pelvis.

If any of these tests indicate a possible pelvic tilt or unevenness of the back, check with your physician.

THE KRAUS-WEBER TESTS FOR MUSCLE STRENGTH AND FLEXIBILITY

Dr. Hans Kraus, a back consultant to such notables as President John F. Kennedy and Arthur Godfrey, and his colleague, Dr. Sonja Weber, of Columbia-Presbyterian Hospital in New York, developed the following tests at New York University to check their patients.

In order to do the tests, Dr. Kraus says, take off your shoes. Relax. Don't rush, don't push, don't strain. Be slow and smooth. Do not warm up your muscles by exercising or bathing before you take the tests. Rest between each test by taking several deep breaths.

If you have back trouble, or any serious health problems, or are pregnant, check with your physician before taking the tests. If you feel pain at any time while taking the tests, stop doing them and do not take further tests or do back exercises without first checking with your doctor.

1. Lie flat on your back on the floor, hands clasped behind your neck, legs straight and touching. Keep your knees straight and lift your feet ten inches above the floor.

2. Lie flat on the floor again, hands clasped behind your neck. Have someone hold down your legs by grasping the ankles, or hook your ankles under a heavy chair that won't topple. Roll up into a sitting position.

3. Lie flat on the floor, hands behind your neck, knees bent, heels close to your buttocks. Have someone hold your ankles down. Roll up into a sitting position.

4. Lie on your stomach, a pillow under your abdomen, clasp hands behind your neck. Have someone hold the lower half of your body steady by placing one hand in the small of your back and the other on your ankles. Lift your trunk and hold for ten seconds.

5. Stay on your stomach, fold your arms under your head, the pillow still under your abdomen. Have someone hold your back steady with both hands. Now lift your legs up, with your knees straight, and hold for ten seconds.

6. Stand up straight, feet together, touch the floor with fingertips without bending your knees.

If you passed all six tests, says Dr. Kraus, you are meeting the minimum levels of muscular fitness and have sufficient strength and flexibility for your weight and height. However, if you failed even one of the six tests, or had difficulty with them, you should consider yourself below par and should work to get in better shape. Otherwise, says Dr. Kraus, the odds are excellent that you will suffer from back pain in the future.

23 CLUES TO MUSCLE IMBALANCE THAT COULD MEAN FUTURE BACK PROBLEMS

In many people the muscles are shorter or tighter on one side of the body, throwing the body a tiny bit off balance. The condition is called muscle imbalance and can lead to pains in the legs, knees, thighs, back, or neck.

Look through the following checklist of clues that might mean you could have muscle imbalance.

• Do you sometimes have to have slacks altered because one pants leg is a little too long?

• Does your slip or tee-shirt tend to slip off one shoulder more than the other?

• Is one hip larger than the other, sometimes requiring alteration of clothes?

• When you buy a dress or skirt, does the hem frequently need to be evened?

• Did you have any injury or disease in childhood that might have produced lengthening or shortening of a bone in the leg or damage to a hip joint?

• Do you frequently get cramps in your leg muscles or in your feet?

• Do you stand in a swaybacked position?

• Do you tend to slouch or be round-shouldered?

• Have you ever had a dislocated joint, a stress fracture of the leg or foot, or a charleyhorse or other pulled muscle?

• Did you have trouble learning to walk or did you walk on your toes for a long time when learning?

• Did your feet ever turn in, or when you were a child did you stumble or fall over your own feet?

• Did you avoid sports when you were a child because you were so poorly coordinated?

• Does one or both feet turn in or out when you walk?

• Do you have bowlegs or knock-knees on one or both sides?

• Do you have bunions, painful heel spurs, or thick calluses where your shoes rub your feet?

• Does one shoulder tend to be higher than the other?

• Are you restless and fidgety when you have to sit in one position for a long time?

• Do you get neck, shoulder, or backaches during long car rides?

• Do you walk with a peculiar gait that others comment on?

• Do you slouch when you sit or stand?

• Do you sprain your ankles often?

• Do the heels wear down more quickly on one side of your shoes than the other?

The Footprint Test

One test for muscle imbalance is to analyze your footprints. Walk in smooth sand, or wet your feet thoroughly and walk on newspapers, and compare them with the following diagrams.

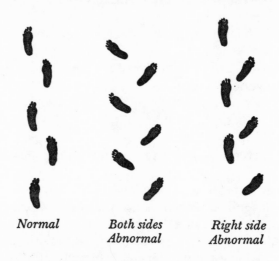

| *Normal* | *Both sides* *Abnormal* | *Right side* *Abnormal* |

More tests to help determine the specific diagnosis of what might be causing back problems when you know something has gone wrong are described in a later chapter.

TESTING INFANTS AND YOUNG CHILDREN

A thorough physical examination should be made by a doctor on every baby at birth, every month for the first few months, every three or four months until the age of two, then about every six months. At each of these examinations the doctor should check the child's muscles and bones to determine how they are developing. Some of these tests can also be done at home as a double check for warning signs that something could be wrong and should be investigated further. Obviously you will do these tests *very* gently and carefully, never forcing motion.

Check your infant to see if one joint seems stiffer than others or if one arm or leg is still bent while the other is completely extended. (In the first few weeks of a newborn's life, do not worry if arms and legs seem stiff and won't extend completely. This is normal; they will loosen up gradually.)

Check to see if there is any swelling, pain, redness, or heat at any place.

Look for any tightness of the skin, especially around creases. All skin folds should be supple and move freely over the underlying bone or muscle.

Compare the legs to make sure they are the same size and the same length.

Look at the spine to see if there is any crookedness.

Examine the spine for tufts or patches of hair, dimples or holes in the skin, discoloration or blank spaces. Whether the dimple is small, whether there is a large patch of long silky hair or only a few tufts, it can be a sign of serious trouble in the spinal cord beneath.

With the baby lying on its back, check the folds and creases of the thighs to see if they are equal and even. Turn the baby over on the stomach and check the creases in the back also.

Place your hands around the baby's sides and hold the infant in the air. Check if the legs and feet hang normally and equally, or if one leg seems shorter or more bent than the other.

If a child is old enough to stand or is walking, you can also check other things.

See if the feet and legs are spread wide apart as though needed for extra support.

See if the feet are turned outward or inward.

Check if the knees turn in or out, or if the legs are extremely bowed (all infants are normally somewhat bowlegged).

See if there is an exaggerated curve in the back.

Have the child bend over and touch the toes, and check for an S curve in the spine or if one shoulder blade sticks up more than the other.

If you find any of these signs, you should get in touch with your doctor even before the child's next checkup.

4 Instant Techniques to Relieve Sudden Back Pain

Perhaps you didn't really need the tests in the previous chapter—you know your back hurts *now*. Perhaps you just started hurting or the pain is occurring more often and you are going to make an appointment with your doctor, but you want something you can do right now for first aid and fast relief.

So right up front in this chapter we give you some instant helpers for your aching back. They will ease your back when you have typed too long, overworked in the garden, or otherwise stressed your back.

But we caution that these are only Band-Aid measures to help temporarily. To keep painful attacks from happening again, to strengthen your back so nagging aches now won't become excruciating pain later, you need to follow the entire Better Back Program outlined in the rest of the book.

FIVE FAST EXERCISES FOR QUICK RELIEF AS SOON AS YOUR BACK STARTS HURTING

These exercises are not designed to build up strength of the back muscles, as are the exercises in our ten-week program, but they are designed to relax muscles and give relief when you are actually experiencing an attack of back pain. See which ones give you the most relief, then do them as many times a day as necessary to gain relief.

1. Lie flat on your back with knees bent and feet flat on the

18

floor a foot or so from your buttocks. Pull in your abdominal muscles, then pull in your buttock muscles so your back flattens against the floor. Relax. Repeat 10 times. Staying in the same position, roll one knee gently and easily out and to the side and back up to its original position. Do 10 times with one leg, then 10 times with the other leg. Repeat if necessary. Relax again, letting your back flatten against the floor.

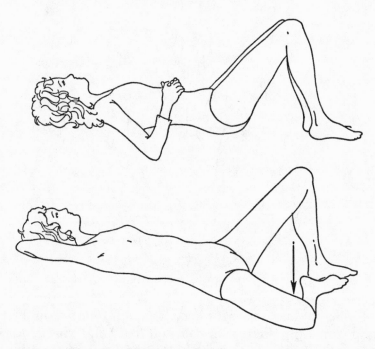

2. In the same position, gently pull one knee up to your chest with both hands. Do 10 times in little gentle pulls. Repeat with the other leg 10 times.

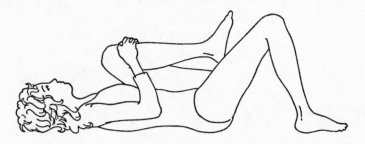

3. Sitting or standing, put your arms behind your back, clasping your hands together. Keep your arms straight, squeeze your shoulder blades together as hard as you can, and try to make your elbows touch. Hold to the count of 5. Relax and wiggle your shoulders. This stretches vertebrae, takes pressure off nerves, and relieves tension.

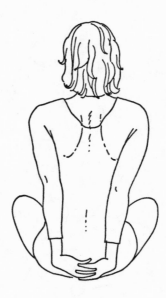

4. Lie on the floor, right knee bent, left foot flat on the floor. Grasp your right ankle with your left hand and grasp your knee with your right hand. With the heel turned toward the groin, pull ankle and knee gently toward the chest. Hold for a count of 10. Repeat with the other leg. This exercise can also be done while sitting, if that is more comfortable for you.

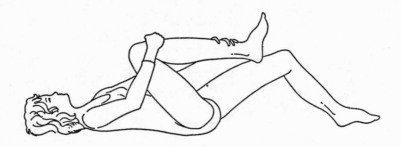

5. In a sitting position again, grab your right ankle with your left hand, place your right heel at your left knee. With your right hand, push your right knee down toward the floor gently 10 times. Repeat with the other knee.

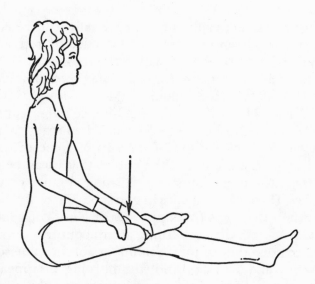

HELP FROM A SLANT BOARD

Lying feet up, head down on a slant board can help the spine straighten out and the back flatten. The blood flows from the feet and legs, easing blood vessels and getting rid of congestion or swelling. Muscles relax. Sagging abdominal muscles get a lift.

You can buy a slant board, or make one yourself by using any suitable large board (such as an ironing board) or a piece of plywood and propping it up firmly on something so that your feet are a foot or so higher than your head.

TRY HEAT

Most doctors feel that heat is useful in easing discomfort and promoting relaxation. Almost any form of heat can be used—a hot water bottle, heating pad, heat lamp, hot towels wrapped in a dry towel to prevent scalding, or simply soaking in a hot tub or shower. However, some doctors feel heat is a mistake, that the inflamed muscles are already congested and heat brings more blood and congestion which the muscle doesn't need. Test for yourself whether heat makes you feel better or worse.

TRY ICE

Ice often works better than heat. Especially if there is muscle spasm, an ice rubdown often can be effective by returning the muscle to its relaxed state, eliminating the spasm.

An at-home ice massage. This technique is recommended by the Department of Rehabilitation Medicine at New York Hospital–Cornell Medical Center. Fill 4-ounce paper cups ¾ full of water and put in the freezer till frozen. When ready to use, tear off about one inch of the top of the cup so some of the ice is showing, leaving the bottom of the cup so that it can be used to hold. Massage the entire muscle area using circular or up-and-down strokes. Do not hold the ice in one spot. There will be a cold sensation when the ice is first applied, the New York specialists said, then an aching, then a burning after about five minutes. At this point, remove the ice for a minute or so, they advise. Then return the ice and massage until the burning disappears, and there is numbness. This is the crucial phase and the end of the massage. Do not massage more than seven minutes in a small area.

An alternative to this method is to use a plastic bag filled with ice cubes. Wrap the ice-filled plastic bag in a thin, wet towel and place it over the area, keeping it in place for twenty to thirty minutes until numbness occurs.

Repeat either procedure two to three times a day, or even every two hours, some doctors advise. When pain is gone, you can gently exercise the area.

MASSAGE

A general massage and a gentle massage of the local painful area can be helpful in reducing muscle spasm and promoting relaxation. Give gentle massage with warm rubbing alcohol or witch hazel. Rub toward the heart. If pain eases enough, you can rub more forcefully, and knead gently to help loosen stiff muscles.

If you want to give a professional-style water massage, you can order a whirlpool bath to fit over the side of a standard bathtub. (Available from Everest and Jennings, 1803 Pontius Avenue, Los Angeles, California 90025, or from local hospital supply houses.) Everest and Jennings also has a moist heat treatment pad called Therm-O-Lax that produces a layer of moisture between the heating unit and the body, when moist heat is recommended.

TRY A CORSET

A well-fitted corset twelve to fifteen inches high is sometimes helpful to give support and relieve discomfort. However, doctors warn that corsets should be worn *only* as a temporary measure and should be discarded as soon as acute pain is gone; then back-strengthening exercises should begin.

HOW TO TAPE THE BACK

Sometimes the back can be given support by strapping. Someone will have to help you. Do it as follows:

Bare your back from the tailbone up. Have your helper cover the back area to be taped with tincture of benzoin or Pre-tac, obtainable at your drugstore.

If there is a great deal of body hair, shave it off so tape removal later doesn't pull hairs.

Cut six pieces of three-inch tape in strips about twelve to fifteen inches long.

Starting at the lowest part of the back, stick on tape horizontally, extending it well across the back.

Lay each strip a half inch higher on the back, overlapping as you go.

Mold tape to the back with warm hands.

Keep in place five to seven days, or remove sooner if pain is gone.

PAIN-RELIEVER MEDICINES

Aspirin (two tablets every four to six hours is most commonly recommended) is especially appropriate for back pain because it has anti-inflammatory properties as well as being a painkiller. If pain is severe so you cannot rest because of it, codeine may sometimes be given for a short time. Sometimes your doctor will order codeine (30 milligrams) to be combined with aspirin (two tablets) to keep the dosage of codeine low. Don't take codeine for long periods because of the possibility of dependence. And when you take it, watch out for often-occurring constipation, which can mean straining that stresses back muscles all over again.

WHEN TO CALL THE DOCTOR

If the backache persists or gets worse instead of better.

If you get backaches with increasing frequency or severity.

If you have other symptoms with the backache, such as fever, urinary problems, genital symptoms.

If pain radiates down an arm or leg.

If pain wakes you up in the middle of the night.

If you also have numbness or tingling in your arm or leg or a feeling of weakness.

If you have more than two seriously painful attacks in a year.

If it doesn't improve a little with a day of rest.

If you were injured at work (a doctor's statement is required for Workmen's Compensation).

5 Exploding Old Myths about Posture

Faulty posture is one of the most common underlying causes of back pain. It can alter the curve of the back and put severe abnormal stresses on overworked supporting muscles and ligaments. If you have round shoulders, a slumped back, or a protruding abdomen, you probably already have back pain . . . or you will have in the future.

But you are also wrong if you have an exaggerated, at-attention military stance, with shoulders thrown too far back, chest and derrière sticking out, and a deep, swayed curve to the back—that, too, means backache. Doctor after doctor I talked to warned against this drill-sergeant stance which we so often teach our children, because, they said, despite all the old theories that this was good posture, it actually forces too great a curve in the back.

There are only five basic things you have to remember about good posture, and you should remind yourself of them throughout the day until they are second nature.

All day long in everything you do, try to stand tall.

Keep your head straight, not thrust forward or looking down.

Pull your stomach in.

Pull your derrière in and your pelvis up.

And most important of all, and we'll keep telling you this all through the book: *avoid swayback at all times.*

POSTURE TESTS

Stand in front of a full-length mirror in your underwear. Check how you look when you take the five basic positions above, compared to when you slump or stand with a forced stance.

Now stand with your back against the mirror or up against a wall with your head, shoulders, and heels touching the mirror or wall, your back as flat as possible. You should just barely be able to slide your hand between the wall and the small of your back. More space than that means your posture needs correction. If you cannot touch your heels to the wall at the same time your shoulders and head touch, your posture needs even more work.

Now face the mirror or wall with toes touching the wall. Slowly lean in to the wall, keeping your normal posture. Notice which part of your body touches first. If your chest touches first, your posture is probably good. If your abdomen touches first, your posture is very poor and your back is under a great deal of strain.

If you are testing children. Young children often have a natural potbelly, and from age six to twelve they may have a swayback, slightly rounded shoulders, and a flat chest, so do not let these variations worry you. By the adolescent years, however, the abdomen should be flat, and the normal adult posture should be attained.

HOW TENSION AFFECTS POSTURE

According to Dr. Marilyn Moffat, associate professor of the department of physical therapy at New York University, the more tense you are, the more the head goes forward and the tighter the muscles in the upper and lower back and the neck tend to be. All of this tension affects the posture, causing muscle soreness and backache. Keep relaxed, but follow the five basic points.

THE BEST EXERCISES TO IMPROVE POSTURE

Do these exercises when you get up from bed, during the afternoon, and in the evening.

1. Stand with your heels and shoulders to the wall as you did in the posture test and rhythmically push the small of your back

toward the wall to try to flatten your back and make less space between it and the wall. Squeeze your buttocks in and pull your abdomen in, and feel your back flatten out. Try walking around the room in this position. Return to the wall and flatten your back again. Do 5 times.

2. Stand with your feet slightly apart and touch the tips of your fingers together in front of your chest; your elbows should be at shoulder height. Keeping your elbows bent, thrust your upper arms back and tighten your shoulder blades (to the count 1-2). Straighten your arms and swing your entire arm back at shoulder height, with your thumbs pointing toward the ceiling (to the count 3-4). Do 5 times.

3. Make a windmill action with your arms. Standing straight (be sure your head is not thrust forward in this exercise or the preceding one), bring one arm forward, then up, then back and down. Keep your shoulders back as much as you can and make large, free-swinging circles. Do 25 times with the right arm, then 25 times with the left.

4. Lie flat on the floor with your knees bent and your feet touching the floor. Press your back and shoulders into the floor, making your back as flat as possible so there is no space between it and the floor. Do rhythmically 25 times. Then lie flat on your back, resting, while continuing to hold your back flat to the floor.

The exercises in the Better Back Exercise Program will also improve posture greatly (see Chapter 12, The Better Back Ten-Week Exercise Program).

POSTURE GAMES

1. Imagine that your head is a helium-filled balloon, trying to pull your body up, and that your spine is a string attached to it.
2. Imagine you are carrying water with a yoke and two buckets. Doing that should trigger your shoulders into proper position, hanging easily and freely.
3. Imagine you are a kangaroo that walks with a tail draped behind and barely touching the floor. As you walk, picture your tail gliding along like a long skirt. Your "tail" can help balance your weight and smooth your walk.
4. Pretend you are a puppet suspended from a string in the ceiling.

OTHER POSTURE IMPROVERS TO TRY

Don't slouch in your chair.

Don't sit with one foot up under you.

Don't always stand with your weight on one foot.

Keep your muscles toned through regular walking, swimming, or other whole-body exercises as well as doing the Better Back Program special exercises.

Put a foot up on a five- or six-inch high stool or step if you have to stand for a long time. (It's no coincidence that bars have railings. Putting one foot up on a bar rail is relaxing because it takes the strain off your back so you stay longer and drink more.)

Don't wear brassières or belts so tight that they restrict the rib cage and prevent free movement. Make sure bras fit well and offer support.

Don't wear extremely high heels. They throw your body weight too far forward and you have to arch your back to keep balanced.

Don't use heavy shoulder bags routinely; when you do use a shoulder bag, alternate from one shoulder to the other.

Don't always use one hand to reach for things; occasionally use the other one.

Get rid of any excess weight that puts stress on posture.

Wear shoes with good arch supports.

Don't hold the phone by hunching one shoulder up and cocking your head.

Don't slouch because you think it's cool or because you are embarrassed at being extra tall.

When you walk down the street, occasionally glance at your reflection in a store window. If you see your head jutting forward or your back arched, realign your body.

Keep thinking about how the way you carry your body reflects the way you feel about yourself. Feel proud and stand tall.

6 What Doctors Say Shoes Can Do to Your Back

The feet can often be at the bottom of a back problem. *In fact, many doctors reported to us that some one out of every four of their patients' backaches were due to foot problems!*

When your feet are weak, or improperly balanced, or hurt, they can throw the entire muscle structure of the legs, the hips, and eventually the back out of balance, causing problems from neck to toe. The U.S. Public Health Service reports that some 87 percent of Americans have some kind of foot problem, a quarter of them serious enough to be called a disability. (Four times more women than men have foot problems, probably, foot doctors say, because so many women wear high heels and pointed-toe shoes.)

Many times one of the best ways to treat your back is to see a foot specialist (podiatrist).

Both podiatrists and orthopedic surgeons we interviewed confirmed over and over that it's not just how you stand that's important to your back, but where you stand and what you have on your feet. And the more you stand on your feet, the more important the state of your feet is to your back. Surgeons and dentists, for example, who are on their feet nearly the entire day, are constantly looking for ways to help their feet so their feet can help their backs.

Here are some rules we gathered from the experts that you can apply to your feet.

EIGHT WAYS TO HAVE FIT FEET

Buy shoes that really fit. *Insist* that the salesman measure your feet.

Keep shoes in good repair—no run-down heels or other hazards to throw you off balance.

Go barefoot in the house, on grass, and in the sand.

Don't go barefoot on hard city street and sidewalk surfaces or where there is likelihood of infection.

Wiggle your toes and rotate your feet when you are sitting for long periods.

Wear socks ½ to ¾ inch longer than your foot, to allow wiggle-room.

Avoid wearing boots all day. They tax your muscles, bind your leg from toe to knee, are tiring because of the weight, and can't be kicked off easily to rest the feet at odd moments.

Avoid running and jogging long distances on hard surfaces. Find earth or grass paths, *not asphalt or concrete.*

HOW TO CHOOSE SHOES THAT ARE
BEST FOR YOUR FEET AND YOUR BACK

The sole should be flexible (bend it to see).

There should be steel shanks or arch supports that do *not* bend.

The leather should be soft (make sure there are no ridges, wrinkles, or bumps inside to rub).

Make sure shoes are wide enough (about ¼ inch bigger than your foot; the leather over the instep should be loose enough so a little bit can be pinched up). Avoid sharply pointed toes.

Make sure the ball of the foot fits snugly where the arch meets the sole, not forward of that.

Fashion is fine, but don't be a fashion plate at the expense of your feet and back. Avoid sling-back shoes or very high heels that pitch the body forward and tend to cause swayback. (Maximum heel height for women should be 1½ to 2 inches, we were told.) Avoid thick platform shoes—they can be hazardous to your health, not only by throwing body balance off, but also by making it easy to turn your ankle and fall.

Try a pair of shoes with heavy crepe soles and rubber heels to see if their shock-absorbing quality eliminates hip and back problems.

For running shoes, make sure there is enough shock absorption; look for shoes with three layers of heel.

Make sure that your shoes are made of a substance that "breathes" so feet do not become sweaty.

If you have leg, back, or hip problems, talk to an orthopedic specialist or podiatrist about whether you should have slightly higher heels than average, or whether you should have ¼-inch heel pads inserted in your shoes. (Don't do this on your own; you could make your condition worse by throwing certain muscles out of line.)

If your feet and ankles become badly swollen frequently, see your doctor. This fluid accumulation can be a symptom of heart disease or some other problem that needs attention.

Test different kinds of shoes and different heel heights to decide for yourself what makes your feet and back feel best. If you find a supershoe that fits just right and is comfortable forever, stay with that brand and style and the store that carries it.

If necessary, have your shoes custom-made.

Tips from Dr. Charles R. Turchin, podiatrist to the Lyndon B. Johnsons. Have the shoe clerk measure each foot separately. (The length and width often vary between your right and left foot.) Buy shoes large enough for the bigger foot.

If you're over fifty, buy your shoes in the early afternoon, not in the morning or late afternoon. In people fifty and older, feet often tend to swell. If you buy too early in the day, shoes will be too tight; buy too late, and they will be too loose in the morning. And remember that, with age, your feet become less firm and may spread out so they no longer fit properly into your old shoes.

What about sneakers? Is it all right to wear sneakers or isn't it? Dr. Morton Walker, of Stamford, Connecticut, a former podiatrist now full-time medical writer, reports that he tried to settle the question by polling some 500 podiatrists in fifteen states. Conclusion: Sneakers apparently don't cause foot problems, but they don't prevent them either. Biggest problem seems to occur if they are worn all day on hard, unyielding surfaces, such as concrete or tile floors. On earth or other soft surfaces, sneakers permit the feet to flex and bend, which is beneficial.

In general, says Dr. Walker, "If your child has healthy feet, he or she may wear sneakers; if he or she has weak feet, sneakers should be worn only for limited periods of time and only if they have extra support from a steel shank and stiff counter, or are made of leather."

What You Should Know If You Wear High Heels

As the height of women's shoes goes up so does the incidence of foot and consequent back problems, according to Dr. Vert Mooney, chairman of orthopedic surgery at the University of Texas Southwestern Medical School.

"Foot deformities and pain caused by improper shoes are a significant public health problem," Dr. Mooney says. "For example, as a result of the irrational shoes they wear, women undergo forty times more bunion surgery than men.

"It's a shame that more emphasis isn't put on preventing foot problems, especially now that we are in an era of more patient responsibility for their own disabilities."

He notes that in recent years women's shoes were getting more reasonable—wider in the toe and lower in the heel. But current fashions have renewed the push for narrow-toed high-heeled shoes. He urges women not to give in to the phony fashions created just to sell more shoes.

"You can resolve a fair amount of back pain in women by having them change to a more reasonable, lower heel," says Mooney.

Dr. Monroe Jacobs, president of the Podiatry Association of New York, agrees. High heels throw off your entire body balance, he says, contribute to swayback, and are easily caught on a curb or step, causing back injury. In fact, says Dr. Jacobs, "The sudden stop from a heel jammed into a crack in the sidewalk is similar to the jolt in a skiing accident."

If you wear high heels constantly, he says, it can also cause the Achilles' tendon in the back of the legs to shorten, leading to pain in the calves and back.

WARNING ON WEDGES AND PADS

Dr. Arthur Michele, New York orthopedic surgeon, warns people to be careful in using shoe comfort devices without a professional consultation. Many people with tired or aching feet notice that the heels of their shoes are worn down on one side and so buy special wedges or pads for their shoes to correct the problem. "What they may find," says Dr. Michele, "is that their feet hurt less, but their backs hurt more." The wearing-down may have been a warning of a body imbalance that should be checked by an orthopedist and corrected professionally. Even if a podiatrist or physican puts in wedges, always watch carefully for a few weeks to see if both your feet and back are improved, or if you have any unwanted repercussions.

THE SHORT-LEG SYNDROME

In many people one leg is shorter than the other. It may be such a slight difference that you are not even aware of it, but only a quarter-inch difference between the right and left legs can tilt the pelvis just enough to affect the spine and work the muscles harder on one side of the back to compensate for the difference. The strain causes a backache that can become worse and worse with the years.

This was part of President John Kennedy's problem with his back, and he wore a lift in one shoe to compensate for his one short leg.

When you have an examination by your doctor for backache, be sure that he measures the length of your legs and checks for any tilting of the spine or pelvis.

FALLEN ARCHES

Weak arches, fallen arches, flat feet—whatever you call it—can lead to tiredness and aching in the legs and pain in the lower back. With time, they can lead to crippling arthritis of the feet.

If you suspect you have fallen arches, check the following points: You probably have fallen arches if your feet are completely flat on the bottom and no arch is visible on the side, or if, when you look at the backs of your feet in the mirror, they seem to bow inward and appear only straight when you stand on the outer margins of your feet.

You can also do the wet-newspaper test: Walk with wet feet on newspapers and look at the footprints you made. If you have no curve on the inner side of each footprint, you probably have flat feet.

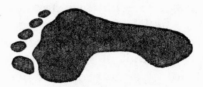

A normal foot

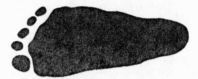

Fallen arch

What to do. If you are overweight, lose weight to take the strain off your feet.

Wear properly fitted shoes.

See a podiatrist for protective arch supports, special heels, and custom supporting molds to conform exactly to your needs and fit in the shoes.

For times when pain is especially bad, elevate your feet and apply hot packs, have your feet taped for extra support, use a warm whirlpool bath, and have your feet massaged or manipulated by a podiatrist.

WHAT A FOOT SPECIALIST CAN DO FOR YOUR BACK

If your back hurts, or if your feet hurt now and you think your back may hurt later, consider seeing a podiatrist as part of the team to give you a strong back. (The old name for a podiatrist was chiropodist, which some practitioners still use. Practitioners attend four years of professional school after at least two years of college, graduate with a Doctor of Podiatric Medicine, DPM, and are licensed by state-board licensing examinations.)

The podiatrist will assess your condition and treat any foot strain. This could include using whirlpool baths, ultra-sound waves, electrical current, massages, manipulation of the feet, and corrective padding or arch supports.

Then he or she will start you on a program to get your feet properly balanced so you can walk with an even gait and avoid the imbalances that caused the foot strain in the first place. For this, he or she may use paddings, lifts, outer or inner wedges under your sole to make easy and correct walking possible. Exercises to strengthen the muscles of the feet may also be prescribed.

SPECIAL FOOT EXERCISES

The stronger and more flexible your feet are, the more they will be able to ease the shock delivered to your spine with every step you take each day. If your feet are one of the body weaknesses contributing to your back pain, strengthen them by doing these special exercises recommended by Dr. Morton Walker for a few moments every day.

1. Walk on the outer edges of your feet in little steps across the room and back.

2. Stand stiff-kneed with the legs crossed—like a scissors—with the feet slightly apart and the weight of the body evenly distributed on both feet. Hold this position for one minute and reverse feet.

7   How to Sleep for a Better Back

We spend about one third of our lives in bed and sometimes another third sitting in chairs, cars, or airplanes. It's no wonder that beds and chairs are important to our backs.

In the pages that follow you will find advice on the best sleeping and sitting equipment for your back, gathered from experts all over the world.

BEST SLEEPING POSITIONS FOR A STRONGER BACK

Use a pillow the right size for you—not so thick that it raises your head and neck and not so thin that your neck slopes downward. The goal is to have your neck follow your spine in a straight, level line. One friend of mine found taking half the stuffing from his pillow got rid of a backache he had had for four years.

Don't sleep on your stomach. It increases swayback and twists the neck.

Don't sleep on soft, sagging mattresses and box springs, or on one that holds your body in a groove that prevents you from turning freely in your sleep.

The best sleeping position: Lie on your side in the fetal position with hips and knees bent, arms in front of you, with your body partially curled. Some people also like to have a pillow between their knees in this position.

If you want to sleep on your back, put a rolled-up blanket or pillow under your knees so your legs are flexed instead of straight.

When you can't get to sleep except on your stomach, put a pillow under your abdomen.

HOW TO CHOOSE THE BEST BED AND MATTRESS

What makes a "good" mattress? One that is designed to support your body weight evenly and efficiently and to keep your spine in correct alignment. It should provide body support and comfort and should adjust to the body contours.

Nearly every mattress manufacturer makes mattresses in various degrees of firmness. Most of us should choose a medium or firm mattress. If you have back problems, consult your physician about the kind of mattress he recommends for your back. Some manufacturers even have a special foundation with a bedboard built in for maximum firmness. Before you purchase a mattress, be sure to lie down on the samples in the store where you plan to buy. See how each mattress feels when you lie on your back and on your side.

Talk to the salesman. Ask him to explain the construction of the mattress you are considering buying; ask him to show you a cut-away version of various mattresses; ask for his recommendations.

If two people sleep in your bed, get one wider than a double bed, which only allows the same width per person as a crib.

Make sure that bed frames are sturdy and fit box springs and mattresses properly. Frames for double beds can be converted to queen size with extension rails. When using a queen size, be sure there is a rigid steel center support bar to help distribute the weight of the mattress and prevent sagging. The king-size mattress rests on two frames for better support and ease in moving for cleaning. The frames can be locked together to prevent them from sliding around. Twin beds also can be placed together with a locking device in the center that easily unlocks for making beds.

How long should a mattress last? Usually, with good care, about fifteen years, so it is worth a little extra money. It adds up to only pennies a night.

Although your mattress shouldn't be so soft that your body sags, it shouldn't be *too* firm for your needs either. Some people find a firm mattress *contributes* to back and neck stiffness. If you wake in the morning feeling refreshed and without any stiffness or backache, your mattress is probably fine.

Mattress sizes. King: 76 x 80 inches; California king: 72 x 84 inches; queen: 60 x 80 inches; double: 53 x 75 inches; twin: 38 x 75 inches; extra-long twin (longboy): 38 x 80 inches. The extra inches of the king or queen can make a big difference in comfort in sleeping and allow for the normal motion of turning and moving during the night that helps keep muscles from becoming cramped.

HOW TO CARE FOR A MATTRESS TO GIVE IT A LONGER AND BETTER LIFE

One major mattress manufacturer gives this advice:

Turn and rotate a new innerspring mattress once a month during the first six months of use. This helps distribute the pressure on the coils so they can give support evenly. After this initial period, turn and rotate the mattress every three months.

Vacuum the mattress and foundation several times a year. The amount of soot or dirt in a community determines the need to vacuum.

Use a mattress pad.

Spot-clean stains on the mattress with mild soap and water; never use cleaning fluid.

Air the mattress regularly. This helps to keep the mattress fresh and odor-free.

IF YOU WANT TO TEST HOW A FIRM MATTRESS WOULD FEEL

Slide a bedboard or a large piece of plywood (use ¾-inch plywood; ½-inch is too thin and will sag) under the mattress, on top of the box spring.

Many people find sleeping with a bedboard relieves the need for a firmer mattress.

If you are staying in a hotel and are used to a bedboard, ask the hotel to supply one. They are usually available.

Haven't got a bedboard? Take the mattress off the bed, put it on the floor, and try sleeping that way.

WHAT ABOUT WATERBEDS?

Some people claim that waterbeds make their backs feel better than do conventional mattresses. The only way to find out is to test one. Rent one, buy one on trial, sleep on one at a friend's house, or get a hotel room with a waterbed.

Waterbeds, like conventional mattresses, have different degrees of firmness, depending on the amount of water put in them. Some companies have air chambers in the mattress to eliminate water motion and to lighten the weight of the unit.

You should also consider the new beds made of gel filling instead of water, as well as those filled with air, to see how they affect your back. Again, no matter what other people claim for their backs, you have to try it for yourself. What is good for one person is not necessarily the best for another.

Here are some advantages claimed by nurses and doctors for water, gel, and air mattresses: newborn babies sleeping on them rest better, are more content, and gain weight more quickly; postoperative back patients are more comfortable; long-term bedridden patients using them have fewer bedsores and less constipation.

Note: If you have a waterbed that seems close to the floor, be careful when you get out of it. Some people with very weak backs can strain muscles simply from the exertion of standing suddenly from a low position.

SPECIAL SLEEPING PILLOWS FOR PATIENTS WITH NECK PROBLEMS

A therapeutic pillow to help alleviate pain from neck problems by ensuring proper neck posture while sleeping has been developed by Dr. Lionel A. Walpin, clinical director of physical medicine and rehabilitation at Cedars-Sinai Medical Center in Los Angeles. He tested more than a hundred patients who had neck problems and found that when they used the pillow for ten days, most of them reported at least a 50 percent reduction in pain the next morning.

The pillow measures 26 by 16 by 5 inches and is made of nonallergenic polyurethane and polyester fiber. It gives four combinations of head and neck support because each flip side has a narrow and a wide, firmer border for the neck. The head can rest on a soft area or on a medium-firm side.

"During sleep, we are unaware that we turn rapidly and put our heads and necks in poor postural alignment for long periods of time," Dr. Walpin says. "This causes irritation of neck joints, nerves, and muscles, which results in head, neck, and shoulder pain, and muscle spasm."

The pillow is available through RoLoKe Company, P.O. Box 24DD3, Los Angeles, California 90024, and pharmacies, medical, surgical and orthopedic appliance dealers.

Another therapeutic pillow was designed by a chiropractor to give proper support to the neck during sleep. It fits the contour of the cervical spine whether you sleep on your back or side, the designer claims, and relieves pressure and tension and affords increased relaxation. The cervical support pillow, called Neck-Ease, is 14 x 17 inches, and is curved higher where it fits under your neck. It is available from Eleanor Levitt Mail Order, 270 West Merrick Road, Valley Stream, New York 11582.

A variety of therapeutic cushions to use while sleeping, driving or sitting are available from two mail order houses, whose catalogues are offered free: Joan Cook, P.O. Box 21628, Fort Lauderdale, Florida 33335, and Miles Kimball Company, 41 West 8th Avenue, Oshkosh, Wisconsin 54901.

Advice from one osteopathic physician: If you have frequent stiff necks, sleep without any pillow, or try sleeping with a folded hand towel wrapped around your neck, to keep head even with shoulders.

HOW NOT TO HAVE A TIRED BACK WHEN YOU ARE BEDRIDDEN

For a back rest, use a chair turned around, a camp stool, or a board with a pillow propped in front of it.

Place a pillow under the knees.

Try a split bedboard. It copies the head-raised knees-raised position of a hospital bed. Split bedboards with supports can be bought in most hospital supply stores, or can be improvised with plywood and stools.

Place a box at the foot of the bed to prop the feet against.

To take the weight of bedclothes off feet, put a pillow at the feet and drape the sheet and blanket over it.

To prevent bedsores, make sure you get into a new position every two hours. Use a water or gel mattress. (Medicare will pay for purchase or rental.)

To help keep muscles from getting very weak, (1) wiggle your toes and make circles with your feet; (2) shrug the kneecap by trying to draw it up; (3) stiffen and raise your leg off the bed; (4) contract the muscles of your derrière and hold it as long as you can; (5) pull your abdomen in as flat as you can and push your shoulders back; (6) with knees up and feet flat on the bed pull your derrière in and your abdomen in and flatten your back against the bed. Do each exercise 6 times; do them as many times a day as you can.

When you are allowed to sit up, sit on the edge of the bed with your legs dangling, then extend each leg straight out. Repeat several times with each leg until you are fatigued.

As soon as you are allowed to be ambulatory, get out of bed as many times as you can; sit in a chair and take short walks.

8 The ABC's of Sitting in a Chair

Too much curve in the back is the cause of most back pain, so the major aim in choosing a chair is to find one that helps us keep our backs flat or slightly rounded. Unfortunately, most furniture tends to *exaggerate* the curve.

This tendency for chairs to worsen the curve in the back means a desk worker is just as likely, sometimes more likely, to have a backache than is a manual laborer.

The pressure per square inch on a spinal disk is about twice as great when sitting as when standing. This pressure is more likely to injure a disk if your back does not have good muscle support, which is often the case if you are sedentary and don't exercise to overcome it.

Psychiatrists, who sit all day, have a very high incidence of back pain. One study of psychiatrists with back pain showed that sitting properly, moving about between patients' sessions, and exercising daily either removed pain completely or relieved it.

"There is hardly a chair or car seat made that supports the back well," says Dr. Marilyn Moffat, of New York University. "American car seats are notoriously bad for backs . . . they do not allow the body to contour into them. Modern furniture is the worst thing that ever happened to most backs. Those big, low, overly soft chairs are difficult to get in and out of and do not help the back."

SPECIFIC RECOMMENDATIONS MADE BY DOCTORS

The fanciest, most expensive chair isn't always the best for your back either. Dr. Henry L. Feffer, professor of orthopedic surgery at George Washington University, says, "Usually the chair that an office executive gives his typist is much better for the back than the swivel chair he uses himself."

Dr. Moffat believes that there are two kinds of chairs that support the back and reduce the lordotic curve. One of these is the classic rocker, with a relatively straight back, the other is the Breuer tubular steel-and-cane chair with arm rests.

Several doctors recommend reclining chairs. Sitting in a good recliner, they say, is like being on your back with your knees propped up. They recommend that buyers of such chairs ask to be given a one-week trial period to take the chair home and test it for comfort. If numbness, stiffness, or pain appears anywhere in the feet, legs, shoulders, or neck, the chair is not right for you. (In recliner chairs, be careful, if you sit upright instead of back, that the thick padding under the head does not force your head and neck forward, causing strain. Also be careful of any sudden or awkward twisting movements getting in or out of the chair.)

One doctor suggested sawing the legs off most chairs, or not using chairs at all and sitting on the floor instead. When he surveyed a jungle population in India that slept on the ground and sat on the floor, he found absolutely no back pain.

ADVICE ABOUT OFFICE CHAIRS

How can you make sure you are sitting in a decent desk chair as a preventive measure against backache? First, make sure the chair is shaped to give support at the small of your back, say designers at a leading manufacturer of office furniture.

"You should be able to pull the chair close enough to the desk so that you can lean back while you're writing to get that crucial support at the base of your spine," they advised. "If long chair arms prevent your getting in close, you'll hunch forward, bending too much from the shoulders."

For typing, it is best to use a chair with no arms and small, firm back. Any good typing chair should allow the following adjustments to be made:

Back. You should be able to raise the small, padded back up or down so that you get firm support from the small of your back to just below your shoulder blades.

Seat. You should be able to move the seat up or down to adjust to your body size, so that you do not have to reach up to the typewriter, nor stoop over peering down at it; keys should be about waist high.

Tension. When you lean back in the chair, it should give a little, but not much. Chairs that give a lot when you lean back in them are sprung, and are much too loose.

Spine Support Work Chair

Spine Design, an office chair, invented by Dr. Bernard Watkins, a back specialist, positions and supports the spine properly while you work. It comes in four models, Secretarial, Draftsman/Teller, and two Executive models. Available from Unbelievable Arenson, an office supply organization, at 919 Third Avenue, New York, New York 10022.

OTHER ADVICE FROM EXPERTS ON SITTING

• Keep the small of your back against the back of the seat. If you have a great deal of curve in your back when you sit in a chair, it is not right for you. It should hug your back.

• Seat backs should begin to contact the back four to six inches above the seat so that the derrière cannot slip under the backrest, and they should provide a flat support at least through the upper lumbar area.

• The chair should be firm enough so that you do not automatically sink into a slouch position.

• The front-to-back depth of a chair seat should allow your knees to bend comfortably when you're sitting straight against the chair back. It should be low enough so that you can place both feet on the floor with the knees a little higher than the hips, but not so low that rising from it is difficult.

• A chair with arms makes it possible to rest your forearms on the chair and allow the muscles of the upper back to relax.

• If you are very tall or very short, try to find furniture especially scaled to your size.

• Keep your head and neck erect, your chin level. Especially when reading or sewing, don't thrust your neck and head forward or drop your head on your chest, straining your neck.

• Don't arch your back.

• Keep the buttocks tucked under to help reduce the curve in your back.

• To put less strain on your back, especially if a chair is too high, cross your knees, or put one or both feet up on a low stool. A good trick when sitting at a desk is to slide out the bottom drawer and rest one or two feet on it.

• When you put your feet on an ottoman or stool, don't have your legs straight out, but bend your knees.

• When working at a desk, bend forward from the hips and maintain correct head position. Have things close to you so you do not have to reach far forward on your desk to work.

• Use a rocking chair occasionally. It helps relax back muscles, shifts the muscles used, and tends to remove the curve from the back.

• Stand up and move around frequently. Even move around as you are sitting.

• Don't be bashful about doing things that are good for your back. One public relations director for a national organization found that bouncing about on the soft, saggy seats of his commuter train every day from downtown Chicago to his home gave him terrible backaches. He got himself a pine board, one foot by two feet, and carried it with him to sit on every day.

• Sit on the floor sometimes. Several doctors pointed out that, for centuries, the Japanese, who sat on tatami mats on the floor, almost never had back problems (although as they have adopted Western ways, including sitting on chairs, backache is now appearing).

• The kind of chair you sit in not only affects the upper and lower back but also can cause pain in the tailbone at the tip of your spine. Doctors interviewed said they see much of this in their patients. "Slumping is what causes the worst trouble," says Dr. Feffer, of George Washington University. "When you slide down, you put your weight on the coccyx (tailbone), and it gets tender, often painful."

TWO RELAXING POSITIONS WHEN YOUR BACK IS TIRED FROM SITTING

1. Lean forward in your chair and lower your head to your knees for two to three minutes. This tends to counteract the lordotic curve in your back that you have probably acquired, which is giving you the back pain.

2. Lie on your back, flat on the floor, and put your feet and legs up on a chair. For maximum relief, stay in this position for about fifteen minutes. This position is good for relieving pain or cramps in the feet and legs as well.

9   How Your Work Affects Your Back

You can do a lot for your back at work, and it is important that you do, because how you feel at work can make the difference between being miserable and irritable at your job, or relaxed enough to concentrate on what you are doing, so you can come home after work feeling good instead of tired and achy.

In fact, the relationship between the body and a job is so important to good health, good mental outlook, and job efficiency that an entire laboratory at the New York University Medical Center Institute of Rehabilitation Medicine is devoted exclusively to this problem. And many companies no longer just have a company purchaser buy chairs and desks for them, but now have consultants from office furniture suppliers come to the office and study various job situations to make recommendations for the best equipment to do each, and then personally fit a chair for every individual.

We talked to these experts, as well as to doctors who specialize in occupational medicine, to learn about specific occupational hazards and ways to counteract them. They gave advice from their research for nearly every occupation . . . the best way to shovel snow, sit at a desk, lift a baby, sweep and vacuum, and lift things.

Check the occupation master list that follows to find suggestions that can help you at work. It's the most complete list that has ever been put together in one place.

THE BETTER BACK BOOK OCCUPATION LIST
FOR BEST WAYS TO DO YOUR WORK
WITHOUT HAVING BACK TROUBLE

World-renowned jazz pianist Marian McPartland lifts herself up from her hips when at the keyboard and leans slightly forward to protect her hips and lower back. Harriet Pilpel, a leading attorney in New York, walks forty-seven blocks every day to and from her office, pulling her briefcase and purse on a luggage carrier behind her. Dinah Shore breaks the tedium and tension of her studio work schedule by playing tennis every day. A leading psychiatrist, who sits most of the workday, gets out of his chair and exercises between patients.

No matter what your occupation, you can find things to do to help your back and keep in better shape. Check this list for things to help you.

If you are a student, don't always carry heavy piles of books on one hip. Try not to slouch at your desk even though sometimes desks are ridiculously out of proportion and uncomfortable for you. Tell your parents if you notice that your spine is slightly curved to the side instead of straight.

If you are a traveling salesman, don't always carry your briefcase on one side. Watch your driving posture. Take breaks during long drives. Learn to relax between customer calls.

If you are a carpenter, you are in danger of developing bursitis of the shoulder from making the same motions over and over. Vary your tasks so that you do not spend an entire day hammering or using one tool in a specific repetitive motion. Be careful lifting heavy doors, windows, and other items when you can't get proper leverage or have to get into an awkward position that can throw you off balance and strain your back. Take a few seconds to get someone to help you. Be especially careful of pounding nails overhead while perched on the top of a ladder. Try to get in a less awkward position.

When you are ironing, you have the same danger of bursitis of the shoulder as the carpenter because of excessive motion in a limited area. If your shoulder or upper back starts to bother you, use that same iron to do arm lifts. Raise the iron overhead, straight up, then down to the side. (If it's a steam iron, empty the water first.) Repeat 10 times. Get away from the ironing board for a while and stretch out on your back, or do a job that doesn't use the same arm.

If you work overhead, you are also in danger of bursitis, but this time in the back of the shoulder blade near the base of the neck. Reaching out and up to adjust levers in an assembly line, for example, puts a special strain on these muscles. Put your arms down as frequently as you can. Do the iron-lift exercise every day until the pain goes away. If you wear bifocals and have neck pains, it could be that you are straining your neck and thrusting your head forward to see overhead through the bifocals. If you will be working at this job for quite some time, consult your optometrist or ophthalmologist about the possibility of having glasses made with the correct focus for that particular job.

If you are a waiter or waitress, walk with a springy gait instead of a jarring one to lessen shock to the spine. Wear rubber-soled and -heeled shoes, well fitted and with broad heels. Do not stand with your knees pushed back and the back curved, which so many waiters do when standing at their stations. Lift and lower heavy trays with a gradual, fluid motion, not suddenly or jerkily.

If you are a nurse, the biggest danger to your back is moving patients. In fact, the greatest number of back injuries among nurses come from lifting patients. Never try to lift a patient while you are bent over a wheelchair or stretcher. Get help whenever possible. When you have to lift, be sure to protect yourself by first flattening your spine, then lifting with your hip and leg muscles, not with those of the small of your back. Lifting can also be a strain on the shoulder muscles.

Shoveling snow or digging a garden: don't be silly, let your kid do it, or one of the neighborhood kids who is out to make a few dollars. If you absolutely insist, do it slowly and rhythmically, holding the shovel as close to the body as possible. As you shovel, bend your knees, not your waist, to take some strain off your back. Turn the body by shifting the feet rather than twisting the trunk. When you shovel, the strain comes from lifting the heavy weight at the end of the shovel. Lighten this strain by sliding one hand down the shaft and using it as a fulcrum, while you push the end of the handle down with the other hand. When you have a very heavy shovelful, bend one knee and brace the handle against the thigh as a fulcrum.

If you work in an ice cream store, you can get pain in the shoulder, upper back, and elbow from dipping out very hard ice cream. Keep your ice cream case just a few degrees warmer, or dip the scooper in hot water before dipping.

If you are a receptionist, make sure the typewriter isn't too far away from you when you type. If you get shoulder, neck, or back pains, it can be from frequent reaching behind you at an awkward angle. Try rearranging your desk and files to keep from reaching in strained positions. When placing things in a bottom file drawer, squat rather than bending over.

If you lay floors or carpets, your problem is the constant bent-over position. Change your position as frequently as you can. Try to relax neck and shoulder muscles while you are working instead of keeping them tensely scrunched up. Occasionally lie down on your back on that beautiful new carpet, pulling your abdomen and your buttocks in so your back flattens to the floor.

If you are a salesperson, when you are between customers, guard against slumping into bad posture habits. Stand relaxed and keep the curve out of your back. To ease muscle strain and stimulate circulation when standing on your feet, make small, repeated contractions of the muscles in your abdomen, feet, and legs.

If you are a musician or an orchestra leader, your major problem is being in one position for so long and repeating the same movements, using the same muscles. Drummers, for example, tend to develop pains in the shoulder area; organists get lower back pain and pains in the leg muscles. Try to put whatever muscles are getting sore and cramped through a wide range of motion exercises between sets. Raise your arms above your head and do windmill circles. Elevate your feet and legs if you have been standing; take a walk or jog in place if you have been sitting in a cramped position.

If you are a truck driver, use a backrest, and on long trips take frequent breaks for food and exercise. When the job permits, be willing to help load and unload the truck. The physical activity is good to counteract the inactivity that results from excessive sitting. (Be sure to use proper lifting techniques.) If you drive a small truck with a hard seat or poor springs, you may develop pain over the coccyx, the tailbone. Attach a thick sponge-rubber cushion to the seat.

If you are a machine operator who uses foot pedals, you may develop pain in the groin or lower back, especially if you frequently reach for pedals with one foot. Mail handlers who habitually kick mail sacks with one foot may develop the same trouble. Use both feet equally if you can, and if not, return your extended leg to the body occasionally. Stand up when the leg is fatigued, and walk about or swing the leg back and forth and shake it.

When you vacuum, try bending the knees. Stand straight instead of stooping over. If your back really hurts, don't do the vacuuming.

When you pick things up from the floor, bend your knees to get down to the floor instead of bending your back, even if you are picking up a feather or pin.

If you are a gardener, kneel instead of bending over as you weed or care for plants.

If you are a dentist, it's the constant standing and twisting that gets to you. Get a stool of comfortable height to rest on when you are able. Adjust the patient's chair and your work tables to proper heights for you, so you do not have to hunch and bend over so much. Get a patient chair that tilts back so you can work more comfortably. Change your position during operative procedures as much as you can. Wear support socks to help avoid aching feet.

If you sit at a desk a lot, get a chair that really fits you, with arms, if that is convenient to your work. Move around as much as you can. Put your feet up on your desk or on a desk drawer or box as often as you can. Don't work with your head bent forward or sideways.

If you stand a lot, wear the best-fitting shoes you can find. Remember to try to keep the curve out of your back. Try to put one foot up on something. Having one knee bent relieves much strain to the back.

If you are a typist, ask for the kind of typing chair that is adjustable, and adjust it for your best height from the floor and best back support. One model that is carried by many leading office supply firms is called Spine Design, and was developed by a back specialist. It comes in many versions and price ranges, from executive to typing models. If you have shoulder or back pains when you type, check Chapter 8, "The ABC's of Sitting in a Chair" to see if your seat and the table height are proper for your body. Perhaps the typing table is too high, you are stretching your arms, or the lighting is poor so you are bending over to read your copy or straining your neck.

If you work at a table, make sure that the table height is correct for you and what you are doing. If the work surface is too low, you have to bend over, straining your neck and back. If the table is too high, you have to raise your hands and arms to work, which strains the shoulder muscles and upper back. Hands and arms should be comfortably in front of you. Keep things convenient and orderly so that you do not have to reach awkwardly to obtain tools and materials. You should avoid working bent over or with your head bent forward or sideways. Draftsmen and architects are wise to use work tables that are high and slanted toward them.

If you are a dancer, beware of foot problems that can lead to back problems. Dancer's foot is an inflammation or sometimes a fracture of the tiny foot bones. Avoid it by avoiding shoes that are too narrow, squeeze the foot, and put extra pressure on the bones. If your feet hurt, get professional help right away because rest alone will not cure the problem. In addition to buying a wider shoe, consult a podiatrist or orthopedic specialist about putting a pad between the big toe and the ball of the foot to help bear some of the weight.

If you are a policeman, you are likely to get policeman's heel (so are mailmen, waiters, and others who walk a lot on their job). The pain is localized directly under the heel bone. Simplest treatment is to pad the heel using a ¼-inch pad cut to the shape of the heel. With a ball-point pen draw a circle directly on the bottom of your heel where the pain is, then press your heel onto the pad. Cut a hole in the pad around the inked outline, then glue the pad in your shoe. When you wear the shoe, the pad will take the weight off the painful area. Sometimes applying heat to the painful heel after work will also help. Do not let the painful foot go without treatment because you will develop an abnormal way of walking that will soon cause leg and back problems.

When you make a bed, instead of bending over, try a squatting position for tucking in the sheet. Consider having the bed raised so you don't have to bend over to make it. (You will also have room for storage drawers underneath.) Don't stretch across the bed to lift the corner of the mattress on the other side to tuck in a contour sheet.

When you hoe, rake, mop, or sweep, stand sideways with your feet fairly wide apart and use the implement in a left-to-right motion instead of forward and back in front of you, which puts constant tension on the back and shoulder muscles. Don't bend over.

When you wash dishes, if you have a lot to do that will keep you standing in one position for a long time, put a little stool or box by the sink so you can put one foot on it. (Sometimes you can open the door under the sink and use the cabinet floor.) Make sure the sink is well lit; it's a place that electricians often ignore. If the area is well lit, you won't be straining forward to see what you are doing.

If you are with the military, your feet and consequently your back may often give you trouble. In fact, one orthopedic surgeon called the backbone of the soldier the military's weakest point. Back pain is *the* leading cause of lengthy absence from military duty. One reason is that soldiers often get stress fractures during long marches, with dozens of men having broken bones in their feet at the end of a march. Make sure that you have shoes that fit, and if marching gives you problems, check with a therapist at the base hospital on muscle-strengthening exercises for the feet and legs that will help prevent fractures.

JOB FACTORS THAT ARE MOST HAZARDOUS TO YOUR BACK

Scientists at Göteborg University in Göteborg, Sweden, recently surveyed various job factors to learn just what the most important ones were in causing back problems. Back ailments of all kinds were especially likely to occur in persons who had jobs requiring prolonged sitting (more than four hours daily) and in persons who stand a lot on the job. Those with the least problems were those whose occupations allowed a great deal of variation of posture rather than prolonged, fixed, or repetitive positions.

Back problems also were associated with repetitive or boring work that does not require concentration, with discontent over the job, and with frequent bending and twisting.

HOW TO PREVENT BACK PROBLEMS AT WORK

Develop strong back muscles and keep them that way with the Better Back Book Exercise Program. These exercises are helpful to any occupation that stresses the back. Surgeons who stand on their feet all day, dentists who work in a bent-over position, accountants and typists who sit at a desk all day, factory workers who lift, truck drivers and salesmen who drive for hours each day—all have benefited from doing these exercises for only a few minutes a day.

HOW TO LIFT AND CARRY
WITHOUT STRAINING YOUR BACK

Whether your job involves steady heavy manual labor or just occasional lifting and carrying, learn to do it the proper way.

Don't lean over from the waist with legs straight to pick something up. Don't let your back arch. *Never* let your back carry the exertion and load.

The right way: Place your feet close to the object, keep your back straight, and bend at the knees to a crouching position; tuck in your buttocks and pull in your abdomen; grasp the object firmly, keep it as close to the body as possible, and lift slowly, using the leg muscles. Always bend your knees when lifting. These rules apply to picking up anything—whether a box, a baby, or a handkerchief.

Move and lift things slowly and smoothly in a rhythm, not suddenly or jerkily, which puts extra strain on the back.

Hold objects close to your body. A light weight held at arm's length produces more stress on the spine than a heavier weight held close to the body.

Don't wear high heels when lifting; it increases the stress.

Avoid carrying unbalanced loads. Use two shopping bags or suitcases with loads equally distributed rather than one heavy one.

Don't lean over a projection such as a radiator to lift a stuck window.

Avoid lifting anything heavy over your head.

Don't reach to pick up something when one arm is loaded with a baby or packages.

Don't lift if your footing is insecure; a slip or twist can wrench your back.

Never try to move a heavy piece of furniture by yourself. Get one or two people to help you, and work smoothly as a team.

Use a wheelbarrow, dolly, or other mechanical aid whenever possible.

Do not keep on trying to lift an object if you feel any discomfort in your back.

If you have back trouble, don't lift heavy objects. Let someone else do it. And don't ever do weight-lifting exercises.

10 What to Do for Your Back When You Drive

Dr. Jennifer Kelsey, of Yale University, has reported that persons who spend at least half their working day driving are three times more likely to develop a herniated disk than those who don't hold such jobs.

How you drive can definitely affect your back. If you drive a lot, the way you drive can help bring on back problems, or it can help you strengthen your back.

Watch your driving posture; don't slump, and keep the arch out of your back. Use an orthopedic backrest if necessary, or simply put a firm 1½-inch-thick pillow behind the small of your back. Wicker back supports are good because they let air circulate so you don't sweat. The Air Force issues an air-inflated low back support for pilots, which can sometimes be found in military surplus stores. Sit with the small of the back pressed against the back-seat cushion.

Be sure seats are far enough forward so that you don't have to stretch your legs to reach the pedals. Your legs should be bent at the knees. Having the seat forward also means you do not have to have your arms outstretched to reach the wheel, thereby reducing strain on the shoulders and upper back.

Keep your head and shoulders erect. If you lean forward, you'll develop pains in your neck and back.

One driving factor that aggravates back problems more than anything else seems to be the long periods of uninterrupted sitting, whether you are the passenger or the driver. Take frequent breaks, to stop and walk or move about.

Avoid staying in one position constantly. Change your position in whatever way you can; and even better, have a co-driver, when possible, on long trips. Even if the other person only drives for short periods, it gives you a chance to change position, perhaps to stretch out on the back seat.

Avoid tensing your muscles. Be alert but relaxed enough to keep muscles from cramping.

Avoid fatigue by stopping for snacks, or carry food and drink snacks with you to munch on in the car, especially protein foods to give you long-lasting energy.

Be careful putting suitcases in the trunk. Get help with heavy ones. Lift them slowly, standing as close to the trunk as possible.

If you are short and you are going to be a passenger for a long ride, bring along a little foot rest to put your feet on to bring your knees up.

GETTING IN AND OUT OF THE CAR

If you have a weak back, you can strain yourself with something as simple as getting out of a car in an awkward way. To enter, open the door without jerking it *or* your back; open it wide enough so you have room to get in easily; enter sideways; position yourself on the edge of the seat and slide over rather than climbing in crouched over, which puts your back in an awkward position.

Exit the same way, moving to the edge, opening the door wide, turning slowly and keeping your back straight until you are all the way out of the car. Then you can straighten up completely.

THE BETTER BACK AUTO BREAK

Do these exercises every time you make a stop. (Or make a special stop every hour even if you have no other reason.)

1. Grasp your left wrist with your right hand, and your right wrist with your left hand. Raise your arms to shoulder height. Attempt to pull your arms apart for a count of 6. Repeat 3 times.

2. Hold your forehead and push your head forward against

your hand. Put your right hand against the side of your head and push your head against it. Put your left hand against the side of your head and push against it. Lock fingers behind your head and push your head back against them. Do each slowly 3 times.

3. Place your right fist in the palm of your left hand, arms shoulder high. Press as hard as you can, resisting with the left hand for a count of 6. Do 3 times. Repeat with the other hand.

4. Put your right hand on your right shoulder, your left hand on your left shoulder. Rotate your elbows forward, up, then back, making small circles. Do 10 times.

5. Stand at the side of the car with one hand on the door or fender for support. Keep your back straight and do deep knee bends, squatting down to the ground and back up. Do 4 times slowly.

6. Put your right foot up on the fender or trunk of the car, with the left foot about 24 to 30 inches from the car. Bounce toward the car in a sort of fencer's thrust. Do 10 times. Switch to the other leg.

7. Step away from the car. Standing erect, with your arms at your side, swing the right arm forward, then up and back in a windmill action. Do 10 times. Switch to the other arm.

8. Take a walk 20 paces away from the car and back.

9. Have a snack and a cool, sugar-free drink.

10. Repeat any exercise that felt especially good, and get back in the car refreshed.

BACK AIDS FOR DRIVERS

Backrest. Helps ease backache, support back. Can be used in the car or in chair at office or home. Attaches by straps (19 x 18 inches). Called Spine Aid Back Support, it is available at Hammacher Schlemmer, 147 E. 57th St., New York, New York 10022.

Contour pillows. These pillows adapt to the contours of the back and give the spine support. They can be used when driving or when sitting at home or in an office. Posture Curve: available through Body Care, Inc., 118 East 28th Street, New York, New York 10016.

The Back Hugger: available from Contour Comfort Company, 7240 Lem Turner Road L, Jacksonville, Florida 32208.

Relaxo Back: available from Nora Nelson, Dept. 46E, 621 Avenue of the Americas, New York, New York 10011.

A number of portable orthopedic sitting and driving pillows and seats are available through the Miles Kimball catalogue (free on request), 41 West Eighth Avenue, Oshkosh, Wisconsin 54901.

Special car seats. Porsche cars, and one special Ford, have as standard equipment a seat called Recaro, which was designed in consultation with orthopedic surgeons. They are contoured to conform with the natural "S" shape of the spine. Recaro seats can be specially installed in any car.

11 What to Do for Your Back When You Fly

Flying often produces backache because of the muscle fatigue that occurs when one sits inactively in one position for such a long time.

Lufthansa Airlines, recognizing the depth of the problem, has designed a Fitness in the Chair program, with trainer Juergen Palm and the German Sports Federation.

Body functions are known to slow down significantly on long flights, Lufthansa officials explain. "The heartbeat rate drops, reducing the supply of oxygen to the blood, the joints stiffen, and muscles lose their tone. One tends to grow tired and sluggish after several hours of long-distance flying, with the condition often peaking at about the time the body should be in prime shape for disembarking."

The following exercises, adapted partly from the Lufthansa program and partly from the fitness program used by American astronauts on long-distance space flights, will help you stretch limbs and joints and loosen the spine as well as improve circulation. These exercises can be performed in minimal space without your neighbors even noticing you are doing them.

First, tighten the muscles of the left thigh. Tighten to about one third of your maximum strength, and do it rhythmically. Repeat 6 times. Then repeat 6 times for the right thigh.

In the same way tighten the left side of the buttocks 6 times. Then tighten the muscles of the right side of the buttocks.

Now try to tighten the muscles of your back in the same

rhythmic fashion. (These muscles are more difficult to control; it may help to put your hand behind your back to feel the muscles; or you may have to simply move your back about and stretch it to different positions.)

Now contract the muscles of your shoulders, again 6 times.

Don't sit in the seat for too long a time. Get up and take a walk about the plane several times during the flight. Take an aisle seat to make it easier. Go to the restroom, wash your hands, walk back to get a drink of water from the stewardess, walk back and talk to that nice lady sitting alone in the rear, if the plane touches down anywhere walk a bit outside or up and down the ramp, anything to move around.

The important thing is to keep your joints moving through their range of motion, from wiggling your toes to changing your head position, all geared to keeping muscles from getting stiff from being in one position and to keep your circulation going.

THE LOWMAN–AUST EXERCISE FOR TRAVELERS

These exercises were devised by the late Dr. Charles LeRoy Lowman, former chief of staff of Orthopedic Hospital in Los Angeles, and physical therapist Ruth Ann Aust, of Honolulu, after their own travel experience.

"I was appalled at the discomfort people had because they did not know how to handle their own bodies," says Aust. "They suffered all sorts of aches, fatigue, and circulatory stresses because they sat wrong and they sat still."

1. Straighten the body. Flatten the back of the neck against the seat back. Sit "tall." Inhale deeply. Exhale forcibly. Relax all trunk muscles between breaths. Repeat 3 times.

2. Stretch upward. Keep the neck lifted, the chin in. Keep the back straight. Press elbows against seat back until your body is forced forward at least three inches from seat back. Hold as you count 5. Relax.

3. Put both arms on the seat arm rests. Try to bring your shoulder blades together in back. Keep them back. Keep elbows bent. Now press both elbows down. Use them as levers to lift the body. Hold as you count 5. Relax slowly.

4. Squeeze buttocks together. Hold as you count 5.

5. Put the right hand on the left knee. Press as you try to lift

the knee. Press so hard you cannot lift it. Relax. Repeat with the opposite hand and knee.

6. Place your hands on top of your upper thighs. Press feet firmly against the floor. Push on your hands as if trying to get up. Hold as you count 3. Relax slowly.

7. Straighten your knees and extend your legs as much as possible. Press your heels against the floor. Hold as you count 3. Relax.

8. Put your heels on the floor, knees bent. Turn the soles of your feet inward. Visualize grasping an object with your feet. Press your soles together. Relax.

9. Stretch one arm up high, as if trying to reach an overhead light. Repeat with the other arm.

Lowman and Aust say these exercises should be done every hour while you travel.

Other advice from the doctor-therapist team:

DO put your feet up any time you can. When you wait in the lavatory line, rise up and down on your toes. It sends the blood back to your heart.

DO stop reading every half hour or so. Change position and look around.

DO support the body when you sleep. Put pillows under your head and behind your back. Muscle strain sets in when the body tries to maintain its position without support.

DON'T sit in a slumped forward position. It not only causes muscle strain, but also puts an extra workload on the heart.

DON'T wear round garters, tight girdles, pantyhose, or stockings that are tight above or below the knee. They restrict circulation.

12 The Better Back Ten-Week Exercise Program to Build a Stronger Back

This back exercise program was especially designed to be appropriate for both sick and healthy backs. I conferred with back specialists and orthopedic organizations throughout the world to find the best exercises to make backs healthier and stronger and yet be safe for any back.

So many exercise programs offer exactly the opposite of what the back needs; they often don't help the back at all and, even more important, they frequently cause actual harm to the back. In fact, doctor after doctor I spoke to reported that many patients came for help because of back problems caused by the very exercise programs the patients had enrolled in to improve their fitness. They talked of slipped disks from dance classes; pinched nerves caused by weight-lifting; sprains and strains of weekend athletes who over-exert on days off but have no exercise program during the week; even back problems in children caused by improper calisthenics routinely taught in many school physical education classes.

The Better Back Program has been designed with the cooperation of some of the world's most respected back specialists to avoid these problems. We recommend only the exercises that doctors have found in clinical practice to really work in their patients and to never do harm. There are no back-bending or nerve-pinching exercises. And it is a graduated program, designed to be suitable for everyone, from small children to grandmothers, whether in shape or not, because it begins gradually and works methodically up to a more vigorous pace. Because the program is individualized and adjustable, you can always be at a level that is safe and comfortable for you, gaining strength and improved functions as each day progresses.

These exercises are effective enough so that athletes use them. Doug Sanders, the professional golf star, uses many exercises like ours, for example, and Dr. H. Paul Bauer, physician for the San Diego Padres baseball team and the San Diego Rockets basketball team, prescribes many for his teams. Dr. William G. Hamilton, orthopedic consultant to the New York City Ballet and School of American Ballet, prescribes some for dancers. And the exercises are also gentle enough that doctors often use them before and after surgery for back patients.

However, if you have any current or past back problems, you should check with your doctor before beginning the program to make absolutely sure that you do not have a special condition that should be treated in a different manner.

Do the exercises for the back really work?

The very latest research shows that the right exercises *actually can increase bone density.* Two orthopedists, Dr. Nils Westlin and Dr. Bo Nilsson, of the General Hospital in Malmo, Sweden, have found that the ends of the leg bones in young athletic men were much more compact than those of non-athletes of the same age. And, say Westlin and Nilsson, the density increased as the men stepped up their physical activity.

Some doctors even use certain of the exercises in patients before surgery so the patients will be in better condition for surgery, and they use them after surgery to speed the patients' recovery and build up back strength and flexibility again. And many times these exercises do so much good that patients with even the most severe pain and weakness *do not have to have the surgery that was planned!*

But what if I'm strong already?

You may be strong, but your back muscles may be weak. One doctor told us of treating a famous tennis pro who had severe back pain despite the fact that he played tennis seven days a week. "He might be a winner at Wimbledon, but he had poor abdominal and back muscles," the doctor said.

(In more than 5,000 cases of back pain studied at Columbia

University and New York University, doctors found that *tightness* as well as muscle weakness was the cause of four out of five aching backs.)

Why are abdominal muscles important?

Because they support the spine as much as the back muscles do. Dr. Willibald Nagler, physiatrist-in-chief at New York Hospital–Cornell Medical Center in New York City, relates that in the days of the Roman Empire, officers, who were the privileged class, traveled on horseback and, as a result, frequently developed flabby abdomens. Any time such an officer was spotted by his commander, he was deprived of his horse and became a simple foot-soldier again.

"There is a very definite relationship between weakness of abdominal muscles and low back pain," says Dr. Nagler. "The abdominal muscles, acting against the pull of the intestines and certain hip muscles, help to prevent hyperlordosis (hollow or swayback). It therefore follows that weak abdominal muscles cause an overstress on the back muscles."

The strengthening of abdominal muscles has traditionally been carried out by doing sit-ups with the legs stretched straight out on the floor. But such sit-ups strengthen mostly the hip flexors (which are usually strong enough in most people anyway), and rotate the pelvis from the horizontal to the vertical position. A pelvic inclination of over 70 degrees causes *overstress* on the back and hip extensor muscles, thus inviting back problems. "The pressure on the lumbar disks as a result of these traditional straight sit-ups increases strikingly," Nagler says.

Doing exercises that strengthen *the abdominal muscles* instead of *hip muscles* makes the entire back stronger, he says. The buttocks muscles also help flatten and strengthen the back.

How is the program individualized?

It starts at a very basic level, which begins to ease your back muscles into the program without danger. You hold each muscular contraction only as long as it is comfortable and gradually increase the holding time. At first, the exercises may seem so easy that you may think they are not doing any good, but do not be tempted to move ahead without doing the preliminary easy exercises. They are specifically designed to be pleasant enough so that you will continue them.

Some people work faster and some slower, but I find that it usually takes only about thirteen minutes to ease through the exercises.

Each exercise is introduced so that you do it only a few times in the beginning, then build up each day to doing it more times and to holding various positions for longer periods. If an exercise is difficult for you, build up gradually, even extending it to the next week if necessary. If the exercise is easy for you, you are able to speed it up more quickly and feel the benefits even sooner. You always move along at your own pace, and in a few weeks you will be amazed that anything so simple could have accomplished so much.

How often should I do the exercises?

To get the maximum benefit you should do them every day during the actual ten-week program. Later, after you are on the reduced maintenance level of the exercises, you can reduce the frequency of performance, if you wish, to every other day.

You can exercise any time of day, except that you should not exercise for an hour after any meal. Mornings are especially good because the exercises limber up your back muscles for the day and get rid of any morning stiffness. But if you are very rushed in the morning, you may prefer to do the exercises in the evening before dinner or before bedtime.

The important thing is that you have a specific time set aside in your schedule so that you do the exercises regularly. And make certain that others do not disturb you, or schedule other things for this time. Let them know you are serious about the program.

What if I feel too tired to exercise?

Contrary to what most people think, moderate exercising when you are tired can actually perk you up and make you feel better, and it also works very well to counteract chronic fatigue. If, however, you are utterly and unusually exhausted or coming down with an illness, you should put off exercising until the next day.

What if I stop exercising for a while?

If, because of a long illness or some other reason, you do not keep up with the exercises, you should start over again at the beginning so that your body will build back up gradually without strain. If you only miss the exercises for a short while, then you can back up just a week or so in the program.

How soon will I see results?

Within a few weeks you should begin to see some results in the way you feel, in having more energy, less pain, and more flexibility to your back. But it will be four to six weeks before you begin to see and feel any really significant improvement. And for the full maximum satisfying improvement, with greatly increased function and dramatic reduction in pain, you must think in terms of the total ten weeks. It may seem to be a long time, but most people feel that the dramatic improvement in the way they feel makes it worthwhile. And, remember, it took years to get your back the way it is now; you can't change it in one week. You want to feel a real improvement that is safe and that will last for the rest of your life.

IMPORTANT EXERCISE DOS

Decide on one place to do your exercises. Spread a beach towel or comforter, or just use the carpet, whichever you like. You need a firm surface. Exercise with bare feet in loose, comfortable clothes that don't bind.

Have a glass of water or juice before beginning. (Don't believe the old wives' tale about not drinking when exercising; it's good to replace water loss.)

The exercises should be done every day for the maximum benefit and quickest results.

They should be done when you are relaxed, not rushed. Some people find their muscles are most relaxed if they use a heating pad or take a warm shower before beginning. Others prefer to shower afterward.

Do the warm-up exercises each day before you begin the more vigorous exercises.

Do each exercise slowly and smoothly. Use no jerky movements.

Progress gradually at your own pace. Do each exercise only a few times, then gradually build up the number of times each day you do it. At any time you don't feel you are ready to advance to the next level, simply repeat that week's exercises for another week until you feel ready to progress. Doing a few exercises well will produce more results in the long run than doing a large number poorly. Every day your muscles will be getting longer, stronger, and more flexible, and the exercises will become easier and easier. When the more difficult exercises are introduced, your muscles will have been prepared by the exercising you did previously.

If at any time you have pain or significant discomfort while doing any of the exercises, stop that exercise for several days. Try it again a few days later *carefully* and with fewer repetitions. If you still have discomfort, *check with your doctor before continuing*.

Rest a few moments between exercises.

Think about your muscles as you exercise. Feel them becoming more relaxed, looser, more flexible. Feel how your back and entire body are beginning to work for you and how you are developing more natural movements and grace.

IMPORTANT EXERCISE DON'TS

If you have back problems, don't do any exercises that are not part of this program without checking with your doctor first.

Don't do exercises that cause arching of your back, backbends, or anything else that increases the curve in your back. You want only exercises *that help flatten your back.*

If you have sudden acute pain or injury, *do not begin or continue the exercises*. Wait until you have seen your doctor and have reduced the pain or received his approval to go ahead.

Don't skip any of the exercises unless they cause pain. The program is built around strengthening not only your back muscles but also your abdominal and buttocks muscles to support and take strain off the back and add flexibility to the spine and hips.

Do not use isometric exercises unless your doctor tells you to do so.

Do not hold your breath while exercising. Breathe easily and naturally.

Do not move in an abrupt, brisk, fast fashion. You are striving for slow, steady, graceful movement.

Do not exercise right after eating. Do not drink alcohol for two to three hours before exercising.

Do not force your body into painful positions. Any uncomfortable position should be worked on gradually without force.

THE GENERAL FITNESS EXERCISE AND SPORTS PROGRAM

The general fitness part of the program is based on cardiovascular conditioning, sometimes called aerobic exercise. It forces you to breathe hard and break into a sweat, and stresses the heart and lungs just enough to promote the use of oxygen. You begin gradually and safely, then progressively increase both your speed and time, thus always strengthening your heart and lungs, and increasing your endurance and condition.

In the Better Back Program you begin preconditioning your body by walking, increasing your endurance a little more each day. After several weeks, when your body is ready, you may then choose to continue walking, or you may choose another total exercise or sport that your doctor approves for you.

Typical total exercises: hiking, jumping rope, tennis, swimming, running, bicycling, cross-country skiing, energetic dancing, ice skating or roller skating. And there's nothing wrong with brisk walking, said one cardiologist. "Brisk walking five days a week for at least an hour would give you the same metabolic benefits as the average jogging program without as much risk."

In the general fitness and sports program, just as in the specific back exercises, you start easy and build gradually so you gradually stress the muscles, lungs, and heart, and improve their efficiency without straining them.

Whatever you choose, start to do it half as strenuously or half as long as you think you can handle. If you decide on running, for example, start running about half as fast as you can, then, before you get tired, walk for about the same time. Keep repeating the running and walking pattern. Each day build up the total time.

Keep increasing your distance or speed or time, and you will gradually begin to build up your endurance and strength.

Stop what you are doing any time you have cramps, cold sweats, pain or tremor in the legs, difficulty in breathing, a pounding heart, pains in the chest, nausea, or if you simply feel worn out or overextended. If pain or difficult breathing doesn't go away, call your doctor immediately.

To get maximum benefit, you should do the total exercise of your choice at least every other day, according to exercise experts. If you miss any days, at least spend the time walking so as not to lose your improved condition.

Follow this program for a few weeks and you will feel better. Keep it up for the full ten weeks and you will never want to quit because you will feel so good you will wonder how you ever existed as you were before.

WEEK ONE: WARMING UP

The first week's exercises will get your back-building program started on the right road, gradually and carefully. Later you will use these beginning exercises as warm-ups to the more advanced exercises you will learn. Do each of these exercises every day.

Exercise 1. The Body Loosener

Lie on your back on the floor. Tighten your entire body as you take a slow, deep breath. Clench your fists; press your legs together. Hold for a count of 10. Now close your eyes and let your body relax as you exhale slowly; let your arms and legs and jaw sag in relaxation. Wobble your neck, your shoulders, arms, legs, and feet to loosen them up. Raise both arms slowly and let them drop. Raise one leg, let it drop, then the other. Let your head drop to the left, then to the right. Take a deep breath and exhale slowly. Let your body feel heavy, let your arms and legs go limp against the floor, heavy. Breathe slowly again. Slowly lift your shoulders toward your ears, let them go. Lie quietly for several moments, relaxed and breathing slowly.

Exercise 2. Buttocks–Belly Contractions

Still lying on your back, bend your knees and slide your feet about twelve inches toward you. Keep them flat on the floor and your arms loose at your sides. This is a basic position you will use for many of your back exercises. Now contract your muscles to pinch your buttocks together, hold to the count of 5. Relax. Now contract your abdominal muscles and hold to the count of 5. Relax. (Do each 5 times the first day, building up to 20 times each by the end of the week.)

Exercise 3. The Flat Back Pelvic Tilt

In the same position on your back, with knees bent and feet flat on the floor (arms can be at your sides or resting on your chest or abdomen), tighten your buttocks muscles and abdominal muscles at the same time. You will feel the small of your back press against the floor. You do not do it by pressing your legs, *but by moving your pelvis to flatten the back against the floor.* Hold for a count of 5 the first day; build to a count of 20 by the end of the week. Repeat 5 times. (If at first you have difficulty tightening the buttocks and abdominal muscles at the same time, tighten your abdominal muscles first, then your buttocks muscles.)

Exercise 4. The Wall Stand

Stand with your back to a wall or door, with your feet a few inches from the wall. Bend your knees, flatten your spine against the wall, stretch your head up and your shoulders back and down. Keep your spine flat against the wall, and slide it along as you push yourself back up. Hold flat against the wall in a standing position to a count of 5. (By the end of the week hold to 20.) Do 2 to 5 times. Try to hold this position during the day as much as possible.

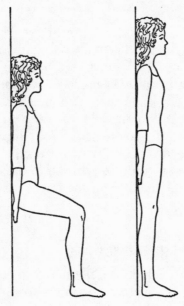

During the Week at Home and at Work

Whenever you think about it . . . sitting at your desk, washing the dishes, watching television, waiting for a bus . . . tense your buttocks muscles and hold for a few seconds. Try to keep the curve out of your back by thinking of the flat-back and wall-stand postures.

Begin Your General Exercise Program

As the part of the exercise program to increase your general fitness, especially of your lungs and heart, take a walk of at least fifteen minutes the first day. Make sure you take a walk every day, and gradually during the week increase its time and distance.

WEEK TWO

Lie on your back on the floor and do exercises 1 through 4: the Body Loosener, Buttocks-Belly Contractions, the Flat Back Pelvic Tilt and the Wall Stand as warm-up exercises. Do each for a count of 20.

Exercise 5. The Pelvic Raise

The Pelvic Raise is an extension of the Flat Back Pelvic Tilt with the pelvis and buttocks actually being raised off the floor. Lie on your back on the floor with knees bent and your feet flat, as before. Contract your buttocks muscles and abdominal muscles to flatten your back to the floor. Now, while the buttocks are squeezed and the abdomen held in, raise the buttocks slightly from the floor (about two inches). Hold to a slow count of 5. Relax. If you have no difficulty, do 5 times. By the end of the week, try to be able to hold the position to the count of 20. If you have difficulty, keep working on the warm-up exercises for a few days and try again.

Exercise 6. The Single Knee Raise

Lie flat on your back on the floor. Grasp your right knee with both hands and slowly bring it up as near to your chest as it will go without causing pain or discomfort. Hold to the count of 5, then return the leg to the starting position. Repeat with the left leg. Relax. Repeat each leg exercise 5 times. By the end of the week work up to 10 times for each leg. You can do this exercise with one leg flat on the floor, or with that leg bent in the knee-bent position used in the pelvic tilt. (If you have discomfort with this exericse or have sciatica pain in your legs, check with your doctor on whether you should do this exercise. If your doctor advises that you need this exercise a great deal, then you can also turn on your left side and do a series of 5, and turn on your right side and do a series of 5.)

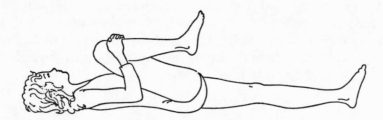

During the Week at Home and at Work

Whenever you think of it—walking, sitting, standing, or lying down—pull in your abdominal muscles and hold them for as long as you can. Keep reminding yourself during the day to keep the arch out of your back; keep it flat.

Your General Exercise Program

Continue taking a walk every day. You should now be walking for at least thirty minutes each day.

WEEK THREE

Do the Body Loosener, Buttocks–Belly Contractions, the Flat Back Pelvic Tilt, and the Wall Stand as warm-ups, for a count of 20 each. Do last week's exercises, the Pelvic Raise and the Single Knee Raise, also holding to the count of 20.

On last week's Single Knee Raise, you can now progress if you are having no pain or difficulty. When you have brought one knee up gently as far as you can comfortably bring it, then very gently rock the knee toward you by gently pulling with your hands with a tiny rocking motion. Do this very gently, and never force this exercise. Start out with 5 rocking motions on each knee the first day; build up to 20 by the end of the week.

Exercise 7. The Knee–Nose Touch

Lie on your back, with your left knee bent or left leg straight on the floor, whichever is more comfortable for you. With both hands on your right knee, bring your knee up as close to your head as is comfortable just as you did in the Single Knee Raise. Now raise your head and bring it forward until you can touch your nose or chin to your knee. (Or kiss your knee if you feel proud of yourself for doing it.) Hold for the count of 5. Slowly drop your head back to the floor. Relax. Repeat with the right leg. Relax. Do each leg a total of 5 times.

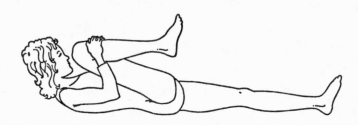

During the Week at Home and at Work

Go barefoot whenever you are on soft surfaces like grass, beach, or carpeting. It strengthens muscles and helps prevent flat feet, orthopedic surgeons say. And whenever you have an opportunity—watching television, talking to your children, reading the paper—sit cross-legged on the floor. It exercises the ball-and-socket joint of the hip and strengthens the hip.

Your General Exercise Program

Continue your walking program. Increase your distance, and step up the pace of your walk from a leisurely stroll to a brisk one.

WEEK FOUR

Do the Body Loosener, the Buttocks–Belly Contractions, the Flat Back Pelvic Tilt, and the Wall Stand as warm-ups to the count of 20 each.

Do the Pelvic Raise for a holding count of 20.

Do the Single Knee Raise with about 20 gentle rocking motions on each leg.

Do the Knee-Nose Touch for a count of 5.

Exercise 8. The Double Knee Raise

Lie on the floor on your back with knees bent and feet flat. Grasp both knees with your hands and slowly pull them toward your chest. Let your pelvis lift; feel your spine touch the floor. Hold for 5 seconds (build to 20 seconds by the end of the week). Return to a starting position. Relax. Do 5 times.

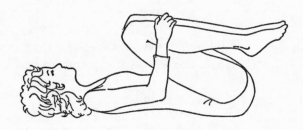

During the Week at Home and at Work

When you wake in the morning or when you are stretched out on a couch, raise one leg a few inches, keeping the leg straight and the toes pointed. Alternate raising each leg as high as you want for as many counts as you feel like it. If you are lying on your stomach reading on the floor, do the same thing: lift one leg a few inches, with toes pointed and buttocks tightened. Alternate legs. Don't arch your back.

Your General Exercise Program

You may continue your brisk walking program for thirty minutes a day, or you may begin a more vigorous sport. Whether you choose swimming, bicycling, or playing tennis, begin gradually. Swim only a few laps. Bicycle or play tennis for no more than thirty minutes. If you are a beginner in these sports, take lessons from a professional instructor to develop proper skills and safety precautions.

Now that you have built up some stamina and endurance and have strengthened your lungs and heart with your walking program, there should be no problem going into a more vigorous sport, but talk to your doctor about what you have done so far, and ask him or her if you may begin the sport.

The American Medical Association gives this advice to help you make your decision. "Initially, walking should be at a speed to cover one mile in twenty minutes. Later the *distance* can be extended to three miles in one hour. At that point, the *pace* can be increased so that the three miles will be covered in forty-five minutes. After that pace is achieved, almost all subjects can progress to jogging."

WEEK FIVE

Do the Body Loosener, the Buttocks–Belly Contractions, the Flat Back Pelvic Tilt, and the Wall Stand as warm-ups for a count of 20 each.

Do the Pelvic Raise for a holding count of 20.

Do the Single Knee Raise with about 20 gentle rocking motions on each leg. Do the Knee-Nose Touch for a count of 5. Do the Double Knee Raise and hold for 20 seconds.

Exercise 9. The Single Leg Raise

Lie on your back, with your arms in a comfortable position. Bend your left leg with your foot flat on the floor, and have your right leg extended straight. Keeping your right leg straight, raise it as high as you comfortably can. Hold for a count of 5. Slowly lower it to the floor. Relax. Repeat with the left leg. You will probably feel a pull in your hamstring muscles. In fact, many people have such tight, short hamstrings that they can only raise their legs to the half-raise position. Only raise your leg as far as is comfortable. Repeat 5 times. If you have down-the-leg pain of sciatica, do not do this exercise.

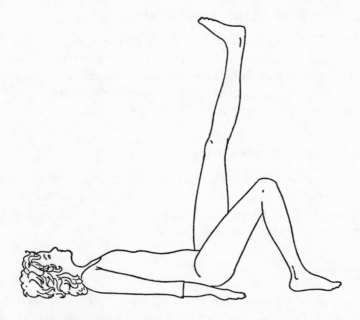

Exercise 10. The Head Raise

Lie on the floor on your back with your knees bent and your feet flat. You can either let your arms lie relaxed along your sides, or you can grasp your shoulders with your hands, whichever is more comfortable. Raise your head and shoulders off the floor, flexing as far as you comfortably can. Do not jerk, but raise yourself slowly. Try to hold for a count of 5. Lower your head and shoulders slowly and relax. Do 5 times. If you have weak abdominal muscles, this may be a difficult exercise for you, but strong abdominal muscles are one of the keys to a strong, pain-free back, so keep at this exercise until you can handle it. As you become stronger, you can come up far enough to touch your fingers to your knees, and the exercise becomes a kind of half sit-up.

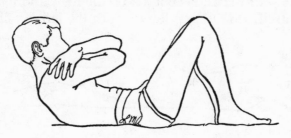

During the Week at Home and at Work

Whenever you think of it—sitting or standing—do the Blade. Put your arms behind your back, clasping your hands together. Keep your arms straight, squeeze your shoulder blades together as hard as you can, and try to make your elbows touch. Hold for a few seconds. Relax and wiggle your shoulders.

Your General Exercise Program

If you have taken up a vigorous sport, begin to increase the time from thirty minutes to forty-five minutes, or until you become fatigued. If there are days when you do not engage in the sport, be sure to take a walk instead.

WEEK SIX

Do the Body Loosener, the Buttocks–Belly Contractions, the Flat Back Pelvic Tilt, and the Wall Stand as warm-ups for a count of 20 each.

Do the Pelvic Raise for a holding count of 20.

Do the Single Knee Raise with about 20 gentle rocking motions on each leg. Do the Knee-Nose Touch for a count of 5. Do the Double Knee Raise and hold for 20 seconds.

Do the Single Leg Raise as high as you can 5 times.

Do the Head Raise 5 times, holding each raise for a count of 5.

Exercise 11. On-Your-Stomach Leg Raise

Lie on the floor, face down, with a pillow under your waist and your arms comfortably relaxed around your head. Stiffen your right leg and, keeping it straight, raise it slowly from the hip. Do not rotate your pelvis; keep it flat on the floor and make your leg work by itself. Do 5 times. Repeat with the left leg. Relax.

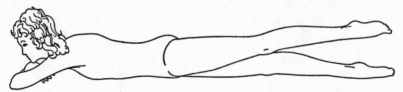

During the Week at Home and at Work

When you wake up in the morning, roll over lazily on your stomach and practice the On-Your-Stomach Leg Raise a few times.

Your General Exercise Program

You have now been on your general exercise program long enough to be able to see a difference in the way you feel. Reward yourself with some new equipment for your sport: a new tennis racket, a new swimming suit, a snappy jogging outfit, a basket for your bike so you can take picnic snacks along on your trips.

WEEK SEVEN

Do the Body Loosener, the Buttocks–Belly Contractions, the Flat Back Pelvic Tilt, and the Wall Stand as warm-ups for a count of 20 each.

Do the Pelvic Raise for a holding count of 20.

Do the Single Knee Raise with about 20 gentle rocking motions on each leg. Do the Knee-Nose Touch for a count of 5. Do the Double Knee Raise and hold for 20 seconds.

Do the Single Leg Raise as high as you can 5 times.

Do the Head Raise 5 times, holding each raise for a count of 5.

Turn over, remember to put the pillow under your waist, and do the On-Your-Stomach Leg Raise 5 times on each leg.

Exercise 12. The Double On-Your-Stomach Leg Raise

Again you will lie face down, this time with a pillow under your hips. Grasp a piece of heavy furniture, such as the leg of a sofa or dresser to help you. Then raise both legs together slowly, keeping the knees straight and the back straight, not allowing an arch to form in the back. Hold for a count of 5. Slowly lower your legs and relax. Do 5 times.

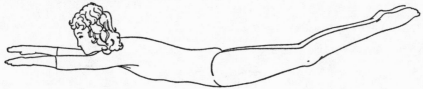

During the Week at Home and at Work

When you wake up in the morning, roll over on your stomach, hold on to the headboard of the bed, and do the Double Leg Raise as many times as you feel like it.

Your General Exercise Program

Invite some other people to join you in your sport to make it even more fun.

Keep walking on those in-between days.

WEEK EIGHT

Do the Body Loosener, the Buttocks–Belly Contractions, the Flat Back Pelvic Tilt, and the Wall Stand as warm-ups for a count of 20 each.

Do the Pelvic Raise for a holding count of 20.

Do the Knee-Nose Touch for a count of 5.

Do the Double Knee Raise and hold for a count of 20.

Do the Single Leg Raise as high as you can 5 times.

Do the Head Raise 5 times, holding each raise for a count of 5.

Turn over and do the On-Your-Stomach Leg Raise 5 times on each leg. Slide the pillow down under your hips and do the Double On-Your-Stomach Leg Raise for a count of 5.

Exercise 13. On-Your-Stomach Chest Lift

Lie on your stomach with your arms relaxed at your sides. Breathe in as you lift your head and shoulders from the floor smoothly and slowly. Hold for a count of 5. Lower your head and chest. Relax. You should keep your back straight and *not* arch it backward. Some people find a pillow under the waist helps keep them from arching. Do 2 times to start; build up to 5 times if you can. Many people find it helpful to steady their feet by anchoring them under a heavy piece of furniture.

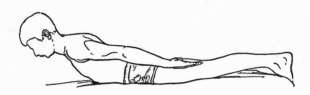

During the Week at Home and at Work

Continue doing Double Leg Raises on your stomach in the morning when you wake up, *remembering not to arch your back.*

Your General Exercise Program

If you have got some other people interested in your sport, make arrangements for all of you to meet on a regular schedule every other day. Practice the sport yourself on the in-between days, or fill in with walking.

WEEK NINE

Do the Body Loosener, the Buttocks–Belly Contractions, the Flat Back Pelvic Tilt, and the Wall Stand as warm-ups to a count of 20 each.

Do the Pelvic Raise for a holding count of 20.

Do the Double Knee Raise and hold for a count of 20.

Do the Single Leg Raise as high as you can 5 times.

Do the Head Raise 5 times, holding each raise for a count of 5.

Turn over and do the On-Your-Stomach Double Leg Raise for a count of 5. Do the On-Your Stomach Chest Lift 5 times.

Exercise 14. The On-Your-Stomach Leg and Chest Lift

This exercise combines the last two new exercises that you have learned. Lie on your stomach with your legs straight and your arms in front of you. Raise your arms, head, and shoulders upward, and at the same time raise your legs up from the floor. Do not arch your back, but concentrate on elongating and stretching your muscles. Do the exercise slowly without jerking. At first hold for a count of 2; then work up to a count of 5. Return to starting position. Relax. Do twice to start; work up to 5 times.

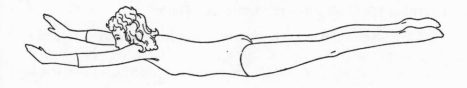

During the Week at Home and at Work

You can do this when you are talking on the telephone or waiting for the water to boil. Put your right foot up on the table or desk, keeping your leg straight. With little bounces lower your body toward your foot, reaching for the foot with your right hand.

After some bounces toward the right foot, lower your right leg and put your left foot on the table or desk. Do little bounces toward your left foot until you feel like stopping. Keep your back straight with no arching.

Your General Exercise Program

Keep up your everyday sport, or your alternating of sport and walking. You should be feeling so much more fit now and have increased your skill so much that you will automatically be increasing your tempo and time just because it feels so good and is enjoyable.

WEEK TEN

Do the Body Loosener, the Buttocks–Belly Contractions, the Flat Back Pelvic Tilt, and the Wall Stand as warm-ups for a count of 20 each.

Do the Pelvic Raise for a holding count of 20.

Do the Double Knee Raise and hold for a count of 20.

Do the Single Leg Raise 5 times.

Do the Head Raise 5 times, holding each raise for a count of 5. You should now be good enough at this exercise to be able to raise your head and shoulders far enough to touch your knees in a half sit-up.

Turn over on your stomach and do the On-Your-Stomach Leg and Chest Lift 5 times.

Exercise 15. On-Your-Back Little Leg Raise

Turn over onto your back with your legs extended straight out, your arms along your sides or under your head, whichever is more comfortable for you. With your legs together, raise them very slowly two to four to six inches, *no more.* Hold for a count of 2, by the end of the week holding to a count of 5. Lower your legs to the floor. Relax. Repeat 5 times. If you have difficulty with this exercise, begin by doing one leg at a time for a few days, then do both legs together. It is important not to raise the feet higher than four to six inches; to raise them higher is actually easier but uses the wrong muscles.

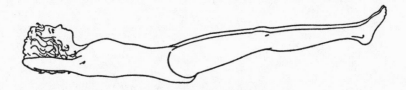

During the Week at Home and at Work

Do this towel exercise whenever you get out of the shower or bath. Stand straight. Grab a bath towel at each end and hold it in front of you at arm's length. Keeping arms straight, raise towel overhead, then bring it down behind your back as far as you can, keeping elbows straight and towel stretched. Do as many times as it feels good.

Your General Exercise Program

Reward yourself again . . . you have now completed ten solid weeks of exercise and should be feeling more fit than you ever have before in your life. Buy yourself another present as lavish as you feel you can afford—lessons with a pro, a great-looking sports outfit, or even a week's vacation to enjoy your sport in a satisfying new setting, and meet new people to share it with.

13 The Better Back Maintenance Exercise Program

Your back should now be stronger and feel better than it ever has before. Now that you have worked to get your back stronger, it is important that you don't let it return to a poor condition. This maintenance program is designed to prevent that.

For your maintenance program it is best to do the exercises every day, preferably on arising, but at the very minimum you should do them every other day.

Keep to your schedule faithfully. If you have started this program because you had a back problem, don't think that once your pain and stiffness have disappeared you can do without the exercises. If you continue to do them and follow other instructions, you may be strong and pain-free for life. But if you stop doing the exercises, your back pain may return.

The Basics to Do Every Day

Since you now are doing only the essential basic exercises to keep up the strengthening you have done over the ten weeks, the maintenance program takes even *less* than thirteen minutes a day, in fact, seldom more than six to eight minutes.

Flat Back Pelvic Tilt (Exercise 3)	Count to 20; do 5 times.
Pelvic Raise (Exercise 5)	Count of 20; do 5 times.
Double Knee Raise (Exercise 8)	Count of 20; do 5 times.
Head Raise (Exercise 10)	Count of 5; do 5 times.

On-Your-Stomach Leg and
   Chest Lift (Exercise 14)   Count of 5; do 5 times.
On-Your-Back Little Leg Raise
   (Exercise 15)   Count of 5; do 5 times.

In addition to these exercises, read through all the exercises for the program and see if there were any that made you feel especially good or that especially helped your back. Add these to the basics you do every day.

After the exercises, rest for a few moments in the basic Flat Back Pelvic Tilt position, and you will be ready for a great day.

During the Day

Whenever you think about it, do Buttocks–Belly Contractions.

Do Little Leg Raises.

Do any other at-home-and-at-work exercises you thought especially helpful.

Keep reminding yourself to keep the arch out of your back, to keep your back flat.

Occasionally back up to a door or wall and make sure that the curve is not returning to your back, that you can keep your back flat against the wall.

14 Exercises People with Back Problems Should Never Do

Do not do traditional sit-ups. If you must do sit-ups, use a curling motion with your feet free and your knees slightly flexed.

Do not do pull-ups, push-ups.

Do not do legs-up bicycle wheels.

Do not do back bends, hip twists, or backward trunk circling.

Do not touch your toes standing with your legs straight.

Do not work out on parallel bars.

Do not lift weights.

Do not work out with pulleys or steel springs to increase arm and chest muscles.

Do not do any exercise that arches your back.

(And if you have weak knees, do not do full squat knee bends, Russian kazatski bounces, or duck waddle exercises. They stretch the ligaments of the knee and impair the normal protective action of the ligaments, making the knee joint more vulnerable to injury.)

All of these exercises tend to arch the back or otherwise put strain on the back, or tend to develop the wrong muscles rather than strengthening back-supporting muscles.

An Alternate to the Sit-Up

The worst strain that can be put on your back is imposed by the sit-up. Swedish researchers Dr. Alf Nachemson and Dr. Gosta

Elfstrom measured the amount of pressure produced by different activities on the disks of the lumbar spine and found that sit-ups caused more than 250 pounds of pressure per square inch on the vulnerable disks, more than the cylinder compression pressure inside a car engine, in fact, as much pressure as a submarine has to withstand at a depth of 570 feet.

Instead of starting the sit-up in a lying-down position, reverse the maneuver and go from the sitting-up position to the lying-down position. Sit on the floor, knees bent, with someone holding your feet or with your feet hooked under a piece of furniture. (You may need a pad or towel to cushion the top of your foot.) Lean back slowly, very slowly. At about one third of the way, hold for a count of 5; continue to two thirds of the way, and hold again for a count of 5; then relax slowly to the floor. This is an excellent exercise for abdominal muscles, but is not easy to do. Do only twice at first, then work up to 5 times.

15 How to Fight Tensions that Tighten Your Back

Our daily lives sometimes seem filled with stressful events that cause constant tension in our muscles as well as in our minds. We read of violence and drugs and pollution and the dangerous lowering of natural resources, of wars and kidnappings and terrorists, and the seething unrest swelling throughout the world. There is often hostility and frustration at work, and anger, sullenness, irritability or boredom at home.

Stress builds.

Your adrenaline level goes up, your heart beats faster, your blood pressure goes up, your muscles tense. Some people develop insomnia as a result, or high blood pressure, sexual problems, or ulcers. And some of us have back pain, because with tension, our back, neck, or shoulder muscles contract, the blood flow is impeded, and we may hold our muscles stiffly in one tense position. It appears to be this *sustained* contraction of the muscles from tension that causes the problem. By the end of the day we may be utterly fatigued, have a headache and a stiff neck, and our back may hurt so much we could cry.

Sometimes the connection between tension and backache is obvious. The tension connection comes because you have been hunched over the typewriter all day, frantically trying to make a deadline you know is impossible, or you have been grimly clutching a phone and clenching your teeth while taking unpleasant calls all afternoon. You *know* why you have a backache.

But at other times the emotional connection is more subtle. A long-term problem may unknowingly be causing stress, tension, fatigue, and backache.

Sometimes the backache is tied into depression. Dr. William F. Collins, chief of the section of neurosurgery at Yale University School of Medicine, says many of his patients with back problems have chronic depression. It's a vicious cycle, he says. "A depressed person naturally moves less and more slowly than a cheerful one. He or she frequently walks and sits in a slumped position. That can cause backache. And, of course, the pain tends to increase the depression, which results in even less movement and worse posture, problems with sleeping, and decreased ability to tolerate pain, all causing a progressive circle of pain and depression that is difficult to interrupt."

"Tension myositis" is what doctors at the Institute of Rehabilitation Medicine in New York call backache from muscle spasm caused by psychological tension. Dr. John Sarno, director of the institute's out-patient department, feels that the great majority of backaches due to muscle spasm are caused by these psychological tensions, perhaps as much as 80 percent. "Most often it's the conscientious, compulsive type of person who's susceptible," he says.

The institute combines physical and psychological help in its back treatment programs. Exercises are combined with helping patients understand that their emotional tensions can cause them to unconsciously brace their muscles tightly.

When the muscles are so tight and braced, even a minor twist or strain can trigger a painful spasm, Dr. Sarno explains. The key to cure is a combination of strengthening the muscles through exercise and learning to relax.

"In fact, I often find," he says, "that the patient who learns that his or her mysterious back ailment may be caused by tension is so relieved that it isn't something worse that the anxiety level goes down and the back starts to improve."

Dr. Louis A. Gottschalk, professor of psychiatry at the University of California at Irvine, said in one study of patients at an Air Force hospital that he felt 96 percent of the backache cases there were caused by emotional problems or were complicated by them.

Dr. Sarno, and all other doctors interviewed, stressed that whether a person's backache is emotionally caused or not, the pain is very real; it is not just in the person's head. You hurt just as much and just as legitimately as if the pain came from a mule kick to the back. And the physical cause of the pain needs to be treated along with any emotional problems that may be creating or aggravating the situation.

Many doctors said that sometimes simply knowing that tension or anger can be the cause of a back episode can help. Then you can learn to recognize when you are angry or tense and learn to relax tensed muscles.

Whether or not they agree with Dr. Sarno's or Dr. Gottschalk's high percentages, back experts report over and over that the person with chronic back problems does often have severe flare-ups and attacks during or immediately after periods of great tension. One study of seventy-five patients showed that the first triggering episode of back trouble was usually physical—straining, lifting, or falling, for example. But *after* that, attacks of back pain were definitely correlated with periods of unhappiness and tension. Tests showed that the back muscles actually became tense when the patients became emotionally upset. The patients tended to be on guard and ready to take action, the doctors doing the study said. But instead, the muscles tightened up, and they developed severe backache.

These patients seemed to contract more muscles for longer times, in more situations, and often unnecessarily. For example, when asked to squeeze a doctor's fingers as hard as possible, the backache patient would grit his teeth, hunch up both shoulders, raise his back, and flex his thighs, and, for two minutes after the test, would exhibit tense shoulder muscles. This use of unnecessary muscles did not occur in persons who did not have backache.

HOW TO PREDICT TROUBLE

Dr. Thomas Holmes and Dr. Richard Rahe, psychiatrists at the University of Washington in Seattle, have devised a scale to help predict not just back trouble but illness in general that apparently is influenced by too much stress. If you have enough changes and the stress is severe enough, it may have a bearing on whether you develop an illness, or when you develop it, and how severe it is. The doctors found that too many changes and stressful events in people's lives—good or bad—too close together often produced serious depression or illness, including back problems. The greater the change, the greater the vulnerability of the body seemed to be.

The life events that appeared to affect health the most were the death of a spouse or other close family member, divorce or separation, jail term, personal injury or illness, being fired from work, marriage or marital reconciliation, retirement, change in health of a family member, pregnancy, sex difficulties, gain of new family member, business readjustment or change to a different line of work, change in financial state, death of a close friend, change in the number of arguments with a spouse, taking on a mortgage or foreclosure of a mortgage or loan, a son or daughter leaving home, trouble with in-laws, outstanding personal achievement, a wife who begins or stops work, change in living conditions, revision of personal habits, trouble with the boss, change in work hours or conditions or responsibilities, and change in residence or schools.

IS THERE A BAD BACK PERSONALITY?

Most doctors interviewed said no, but many did think there was a bad back *attitude,* the way the patients feel about a situation and what they wish to do about it.

Often patients were in a situation where they were unable to act, their action inhibited by others or by their own guilt or fears.

In general, Dr. Holmes says, "Patients exhibiting the backache syndrome are active, anxious, restless people who tolerate idleness and inactivity poorly. . . . They are quick to react to life situations which threaten their security with intense feelings of resentment, frustration, hostility, humiliation, and guilt. They are often unable to give expression to their hostile feelings, but keep them in and ruminate for days.

"They are often neat, meticulous, and perfectionistic, and usually apply themselves assiduously to the execution of any task they undertake, regardless of whether or not it is productive of satisfaction," says Holmes. "Their action patterns are designed to win approval and support by 'doing for others,' 'trying to please others,' 'keeping the peace,' and 'carrying heavy burdens of responsibility without complaint.' "

However, doctors stress that these findings are averages and generalizations, and certainly do not apply to all cases.

CHECK *YOURSELF* FOR HIDDEN TENSION

To make sure unrecognized tension doesn't cause you to have backache or pains in the neck or shoulders, check yourself for these clues to hidden tension. In fact, check yourself right now as you are reading, and then check yourself periodically throughout the day, especially whenever you are under stress, are anxious, are working hard at a problem, or find you are tight and hurrying for no good reason.

The tension clues to look for:
Tight neck or jaw muscles
Tight shoulders or back
Jutted-out chin
Biting or grinding teeth
Tight, strained voice
Hunched shoulders
Tightly curled toes or fingers
Rigid spine
Tight forehead, sometimes with a headache
Sweating palms, feet, or armpits
Irritability
High pulse rate
Brusque movements with muscles tight or braced
Irregular, shallow breathing, or sighing respiration
Butterflies in the stomach
Fluttering eyes, or eyestrain

When you feel these signs coming on, take a few deep breaths and purposefully relax. You don't *have* to grimly grip the phone when you talk, or pound your feet when you walk, or rush headlong, harried and hurried, through the housework. Slow your voice, slow your walk, relax your muscles, relax the fingers holding a pencil or telephone, ease your mind and body into a relaxed approach to whatever you are doing. You will feel the results in your back at the end of the day.

I have found this tremendously helpful in my own life. As a public relations consultant, I used to run press rooms for national meetings, with phones jangling, cameramen yelling, and ten reporters all wanting interviews at once so they could meet their deadlines. There was no way to eliminate stress from the job, but I learned to stop in the middle of a crisis and mentally check for tight muscles and over-reacting. The very act of checking helped keep me from being tense.

My mother used to grimly vacuum, pound up and down the steps to do the laundry, and wash dishes with muscles so tense she could have snapped each dish in two. She found that periodic checking as she did the housework helped her, too.

Once you've set up more relaxed habits, you can check yourself less frequently, eventually only needing to check your reactions occasionally or at special times of crisis.

SAVE YOUR BACK LATER
BY REDUCING TENSIONS NOW

President Kennedy used to lean back on the wall, close his eyes, and relax completely whenever free moments came, even in elevators. Henry Ford said he could handle difficult jobs by breaking them down to small components and working on each in turn. Dr. Paul Dudley White rode his bike and walked for miles. President Eisenhower, when feeling tense before a speech, would picture people in the front row in their underwear. Several famous people use slow, deep breathing and progressive relaxation to eliminate tension. One network science editor hums before going on the air. A famous surgeon sings to relax himself before he operates.

We don't have to have a frenzied, rushed, tense, seething, aggressive, anxious reaction to life. We can *learn* to do otherwise.

Here are some other techniques recommended by back experts, psychologists, and stress specialists to help you reduce tension and cope with stress.

Reduce tension by changing how you see things. Try to keep from getting worked up. Don't meet minor happenings as though they were major crises. It isn't the stressful situation itself that usually causes the problem, it's our attitude toward the situation, our reaction to it. A burned dinner, milk spilled, a flat tire, a bill unpaid, a job lost, a child crying . . . all are potentially stressful situations. How much they affect us depends on the way we react to them.

Reduce tension by organizing your time. If your life is full of conflicting demands, rushing here and there, nothing ever seeming to get done, then simplify and organize. Put priorities on your time and energy.

Eliminate unnecessary tasks. Organize your day for the things you really want or need to do, so you are not always in a frenzy struggling against time.

Keep lists for shopping and for things you want to do. Carry a notebook for jotting down notes as you think of things. At night look at your lists and your calendar for engagements and plan your coming day.

Learn to concentrate on a task when you do it. Don't let your mind wander to other problems while you're taking care of the current one.

Use small bits of time. Watch only the television programs that are really important to you. Use an hour in the evening for a family hobby or to get a small job done. Carry a book to read, letters to write, or other small projects with you so you can take advantage of any waiting or commuting time.

Get help for the less important jobs you can afford to delegate.

Learn how to say no to things you don't really want or need to do.

Try to calm your sense of time urgency. You don't have to rush through every day as if you're running a race. Nobody is holding a stopwatch on you. Take a deep breath, hum a tune, and walk a little slower.

Think about what you really want from life. I remember some close hours spent with Joe Williams, the marvelous jazz and blues singer, and what he would say in his intense way to so many people he met: "What do you *want*? What do you really *want*?" List some specific goals for the next few months and for the future. Try to devote as much time as possible to those goals and to major problems rather than to busy-busy trivia.

Create an environment that promotes peace. Try to eliminate distracting noises and conflicting activities so you can concentrate on what you are doing.

When something worries you, talk it out. Don't bottle it up. Talk to your family or a friend. If that isn't enough, consider professional help.

Escape for a while. Go to a movie, visit a friend, play a game with your child. Then come back and deal with your difficulty.

Learn to live day by day, moment by moment. Try the Buddhist philosophy of paying attention to the here-and-now, savoring eating when you're eating, concentrating on driving when you are driving, not on something else in the past or future.

Pleasure yourself. You deserve a break today, and every day. Nurture yourself. Have a massage, take a leisurely walk, buy yourself a present, have a manicure, sleep late without feeling guilty. Do something just for the fun of it.

Try to find work you really like. It isn't the stress of work that wears us out, but the stress of frustration and failure. Working long hours or doing hard physical labor rarely leads to dangerous tension. One study of 800 executives over a three-year period showed that anxiety was not correlated to salary, number of hours worked, or number of hours spent commuting. But there *was* a correlation between anxiety and whether there was satisfaction with a job or not.

When you relax, really relax. Some people watch TV or lie on a beach and still are tense. Put your problems out of your mind and lose yourself to relaxing.

Allow time for self-contemplation and thinking. Consider religion or read the philosophers. It gives many people a sense of purpose and peace that helps put oil on the waters of stress situations.

Enjoy your family. Whether it's with your parents, your spouse, or your children, you can gain understanding and support as well as enjoyment.

Don't worry so much about money. Most husbands would rather have a loving, understanding wife than a bigger house. Most women prefer a man's tenderness and attention to a fur coat. Most kids wouldn't mind making do with a simple secondhand bike instead of a new 10-speed if they had plenty of love and attention and some time with their parents.

Assess your skills at your job. If you are tense because you feel inadequate at your job, take some courses or read books to improve your skills, or try to switch to another job you think will fit you better.

Talk to your employer. Two of the biggest stress-causers on jobs are not having clear work objectives so you know what is expected and not having adequate facts or tools to do a job. Both could be solved by a non-hostile discussion with your boss.

Try cooperation instead of competition. You don't always have to edge out the other person on the highway or win a discussion. Learn to recognize and eradicate excessive hostile feelings.

Don't try to be a super-person. Give the best of your efforts and ability, but don't feel guilty if you don't achieve the impossible. Be a perfectionist on important things, not on low-priority items.

Do something physical. If you feel pent-up anger or frustration, cool off by gardening or cleaning out the garage. Take a walk, jog, skip rope, hit a ball in golf or tennis, go to a dance, climb, swim. Anything to begin working it out.

Exercise. Regular exercise has been shown to greatly reduce tension, and the physical effects of tension. The general exercise phase of our back program is especially graded to give you these tension-relieving effects as well as body-building effects.

Don't manufacture tension. Some people are always keyed up, tense, waiting for the worst possible thing to happen when things are not really stressful at all. If they don't have stress, they create it. Learn to eliminate tension from your life and you will feel a weight lift from your shoulders, the tightness leave your muscles, and a sense of tranquillity replace much of the irritability and frustration you feel.

RELAXATION TECHNIQUES TO HELP YOUR TENSION AND YOUR BACK

The rag doll. Stand with your legs apart and bend at the waist. Shake your arms and hands loosely. Let your head hang, and sway from side to side. *This* is hanging loose.

Head roll. Drop your chin to your chest. Rotate your head to the right and turn your chin to your shoulder. Circle the head back and around and over your left shoulder to make a complete revolution. Repeat in the opposite direction.

Head tilt. Keep shoulders down. Tilt the left ear to the left shoulder several times in a bouncing motion. Tilt the right ear to the right shoulder several times.

Head lift. Curl your fingers around the sides of your neck, fingers meeting in back. Lift straight upward and forward as though you were trying to lift your head off your shoulders. Turn your head slightly from right to left while you continue lifting.

Abdominal breathing. Lie flat on your back; place one hand on your abdomen and one on your chest so you can feel that you are breathing with the abdomen, not the chest. Inhale deeply and slowly through the nostrils and expand the abdomen without pulling the air up to the chest. Keep your shoulders and chest relaxed, and your back flat against the floor. Exhale slowly through the nostrils, pulling the abdomen to the back of the spine. Some people like to do abdominal breathing with their feet elevated and head down on a slant board.

The sighing breath. Inhale deeply through the nostrils to the count of 8; then with lips puckered (as if cooling soup), exhale very slowly through the mouth to the count of 16, or as long as you can. Concentrate on the long sighing sound and feel the tension dissolve. Repeat at least 10 times.

Do-it-yourself head-and-neck massage. Close your eyes and massage your head and neck in firm small circles. With your head and neck limp, massage the skull, then massage down along the neck vertebrae to the shoulders.

Progressive relaxation. Lie on your back, close your eyes. Breathe in deeply (through the nose); hold your breath, tensing all muscles, then let them go limp and exhale slowly. Now lie limply and take another long, deep breath. Exhale as far as you can, releasing your breath very slowly.

Starting with your feet, tense your muscles, then let go. Tense the toes of your right foot, relax; then the toes of your left foot. Tense and relax the ankles, calves, knees, and thighs. Let waves of relaxation spread into your legs, abdomen, chest, and shoulders; then all along your spine and back. Feel the muscles begin to loosen. Tense your abdominal muscles; relax. Tighten your buttocks and relax. Let your back go flat against the floor. Relax your fingers one by one. Close and open your fists, first your right hand, then your left. Relax the muscles in your arm. Shrug your shoulders, then relax. Relax along the sides and back of your neck. Tense your facial muscles, then relax. With your lips slightly parted let your jaw sag. Yawn. Feel your scalp loosen. Let your eyes relax and rest. Feel relaxation enveloping your entire body. Your upper back is relaxed; your lower back is relaxed. As you breathe out, feel more and more tension leave you. Concentrate on the flow of your breath and feel the state of relaxed peace.

Backache removal hypnosis tape. Self-hypnosis tape gives instructions to relax and let go of tensions in the back. Available from Valley of the Sun Publishing Company, Box 4276, Scottsdale, Arizona 85258.

Meditation. The meditation state is similar to the first moments of falling asleep. It's a quiet state of inner reflection. To experience it, find a quiet place, sit in a comfortable position, and close your eyes. Take a deep, slow, long breath. Let calmness come into your body. Let your muscles relax, your mind blank to nothing . . . drifting. Just let it happen. Observe the feeling of peace and serenity, but don't try to control it.

There are many variations of meditation techniques. With some you let your mind wander as it wishes; in some techniques, such as TM (Transcendental Meditation), you keep saying one word or phrase over and over to keep your mind from wandering.

In yoga or Zen meditation you concentrate on respiration; in one-pointing you contemplate a pleasant object, focusing your gaze on a lighted candle, a leaf, a flower, or on still water, feeling and appreciating its form and detail. Tai Chi combines movement with meditation.

People who practice meditation generally use the technique for ten to twenty minutes twice a day, but not within two hours after any meal. Done regularly, it has been shown to reduce tension and anxiety, lower blood pressure, decrease occurrences of irregular heartbeat, and help smokers, drug-users, and alcoholics quit.

Professional help. Check your doctor, a psychologist, a psychiatrist, a local clinic, or even the telephone book and local university for instruction in biofeedback, TM, yoga, time management, and other techniques for reducing stress. Some cities even have special stress reduction centers using one or more of these relaxation techniques. Sometimes workshops are sponsored by local Y's or health clubs. Some companies are now offering stress reduction workshops for their employees.

STRESS AND DIET

Many people find their diet has a profound effect on whether they are tense or tranquil. If you tend to be tense and irritable, check yourself with these four diet experiments. Do each at a separate time so the results from one do not affect the other.

1. Totally eliminate caffeine from your diet for one week. Do not use coffee, tea, cocoa, colas, or other caffeine drinks, or medicine with caffeine, such as headache pills. If you then find you're less nervous and less tense, caffeine may be something you should cut down or eliminate permanently from your diet. Gradually add caffeine to your diet in small amounts to determine just how much you can tolerate without becoming tense.

2. After you have tested caffeine, try eliminating sugar from your diet for a week, completely avoiding table sugar and all foods and drinks that contain any sugar. If your tensions decrease, eliminate sugar permanently from your diet.

3. Take vitamin and mineral supplements, making sure they contain choline and inositol, the natural tension alleviators, as well as other B vitamins. See if these make a further difference.

4. Often irritability and tension are caused by wide fluctuations in sugar levels in the blood. You can smooth these fluctuations out and provide steady energy for your body by eating a snack of cheese, nuts, eggs, or meat every three hours, or by taking fructose, the sugar that diabetics can use. Also called levulose, it is readily available in Europe and is slowly becoming available in this country in most health food stores and some drugstores.

STRESS AND YOUR ENVIRONMENT

The weather. Many people become tense before a storm. A falling barometer can even cause depression or difficulty in solving problems, so when you feel the weather pressing in, postpone important decisions, drive extra carefully, watch for tension, and prepare for an "off" day. Smog has also been found to be a factor.

The wrong kind of light bulbs. Many emotional problems, including hyperactivity in children and general tension, have recently been linked to people not getting enough ultraviolet light. In one Florida radio station when fluorescent lights were installed, people became irritable, tense, rebellious, and quit without explanation. When UVT lights were installed, things returned to normal. Make sure your windows and your eyeglasses are "full spectrum" (ultraviolet-transmitting) and light bulbs and tubes are "daylight white." Simply ask your dealer for them.

Hidden lead poisoning. Dangerous lead poisoning is spreading swiftly through the population, some doctors say. We're getting it in the air we breathe, from car exhausts, from contaminated food, and even from some high-lead hair dyes. Several doctors told us that many people who suffer from extreme irritability and tension really have subclinical cases of lead poisoning that have never been diagnosed. It can also cause arthritis-like symptoms. You can be tested for lead and other toxic metals by having your doctor send a sample of your hair to a special laboratory for analysis. (Hair sampling is much more accurate than blood sampling.)

16 How to Have Good Sex with a Bad Back

Over and over again physicians told us that the biggest worry that back patients have is whether their bad backs will affect their sex lives. And over and over again those same physicians told us that such worries were needless, that a bad back absolutely need not keep you from having sex.

Some people use a bad back as an excuse for not taking part in sex, but there seldom is a physical reason for not having a full sex life, the doctors said.

Men especially often falsely see a bad back as an indication of a lessening of their masculinity, a sign of weakness. In fact, when Drs. Myron M. LeBan, Richard Burk, and Ernest Johnson, of Ohio State University, studied a group of forty-three men with bad backs, they found that twenty-seven of them were unable to have erections or intercourse—but for no physical reasons! The reasons for impotence were all psychological, Dr. LeBan said.

Actually, sex can help your back. In fact, we will give you four sex techniques that will strengthen your back. Besides providing exercise, relief of tension, and a sense of well-being, sex has been reported to actually help ease pain in persons with backaches and arthritis. One arthritis expert at Albert Einstein Medical Center in Philadelphia notes that many arthritis patients say they achieve six to eight hours of relief of pain after sexual activity.

However, there can sometimes be physical reasons that people with bad backs have sex problems, according to Dr. George E. Ehrlich, professor of medicine at Temple University School of

Medicine, in Philadelphia. The reasons usually fall into three categories: (1) The patient is in such pain that it inhibits sexual desire; (2) there may be physical deformities, such as a woman being unable to open her legs wide enough; or (3) the patient may have lessening of sexual desire as a side effect of medicines he or she is taking. For example, a man may find he's impotent from taking corticosteroids. In this case, the doctor may be able to lower the dosage or substitute another medication. If physical deformities of the back or hips or legs are causing the problem, much can also be done.

"You can be a godsend to many of these people by discussing their problems and helping them overcome their inhibitions about using sexual positions other than the traditional missionary one," Dr. Ehrlich says. For women who have difficulty in opening their legs wide, he recommends rear vaginal penetration or straddle and side-to-side positions. "Or—in the case of a young patient of mine with fused hips who couldn't open her legs at all and was on the verge of losing her husband—total hip surgery, in which the acetabulum and part of the femur are replaced, can restore complete sexual function."

Pain is one of the causes of sexual dysfunction in persons with a bad back, Dr. Ehrlich said, and this can be treated medically. Or there may simply be misunderstanding on the part of one partner or the other about the pain. For example, one woman with arthritis thought her husband was turned off by her, because he wasn't having intercourse with her. But when interviewed, the husband said, "I love her. But I'm treating her like a china doll because she has arthritis, and I don't want to hurt her. . . . I don't want to force myself on her when she has this problem." When they talked it over, their problem was solved.

People with chronic back conditions tend to have depression, and this too causes problems since it often results in a loss of sex drive. Many back patients find that as a doctor treats their depression with medication, their sex problems suddenly are also solved.

EXPERTS' ADVICE ON SEX AND YOUR BACK

If you are having a severe attack of back pain, abstinence from sex is a good idea, but after the pain has subsided, intercourse should be no problem.

A hot bath or gentle massage can be a helpful relaxing and muscle-limbering prelude.

Do not use acrobatic positions that could put a strain on your back.

Avoid violent or sudden jarring or twisting movements, and concentrate instead on smooth, slow, sensuous movements.

Keep the back as straight as possible. Nearly any position is safe as long as you avoid those that keep your back in an arched position. For example, a bad position for a woman would be kneeling with the face down on the mattress for rear penetration, which usually arches the back greatly. Being on the bottom usually causes less arching than being on top.

If a cramp or pain occurs during intercourse, stop immediately, wait for the pain to subside, then begin again slowly in a different position.

Engage in sex when you are well rested if possible rather than when you—and your back—are very fatigued.

Use your back problem to create a better sex life by exploring new positions and techniques and increasing mutual understanding of what makes the other feel good.

If you have had an episode of back pain, resume sexual activities gradually. You can judge how strenuous you can be by where you are in the Better Back Exercise Program. The same muscles are involved, so the further advanced you are in your back-strengthening exercises in this book, the more adventurous you may be with your sexual activities.

FOUR GOOD POSITIONS FOR THE PERSON WITH A BAD BACK

The least stressful position for either the man or the woman with a bad back is lying on the back with the knees slightly bent, flattening the lower back against the mattress (Better Back Exercise 3). By combining Exercise 3 (the Flat Back Pelvic Tilt) with Exercise 5 (the Pelvic Raise), a man or woman can have very effective stimulation and not only protect the back but even strengthen it by the exercise. Stimulation can be extremely effective and the exercise most beneficial if movements are done very very slowly, with the partner on top thrusting slowing while the person on the bottom maintains the Flat Back Pelvic Tilt Exercise

3 position; then the person on top holds still quietly, not moving while the person on the bottom reaches up and slowly moves about in the Pelvic Raise position.

A variation of this position is for the partner with the bad back to lie underneath and place a pillow under the buttocks for extra support and to help keep the back from arching.

In the spoon position, the woman lies on her side with knees bent, the man lying behind her, curling about her and entering from the rear. The woman should have her back in a curved fetal position, not arched in a swayback.

A variation of this position is for the woman to put a pillow between her knees to keep the top leg from twisting and stretching the muscles of the hip and back.

In all four of these positions, the sexual push-pulling, if done gently and properly, will not only contribute to sexual pleasure but be excellent therapy for building a stronger back.

SEX EQUIPMENT FOR A HAPPY BACK

A bed with a very firm mattress and a firm construction.

Extra pillows of different sizes to go under, to raise, to support, to cushion as needed.

A soft extra comforter to keep from getting chilled.

Oil or lotion handy to give soothing, stimulating massages and back rubs.

SEX AND THE PARAPLEGIC

Most paraplegics can have some sex life, according to the specialists we talked to. In fact, a workshop was recently held for spinal cord patients, showing them that spinal damage need not end their sex lives. Doctors at the workshop said that the vast majority of men with spinal injuries can have erections, and if spinal cord damage is not complete, some 70 percent can have an ejaculation.

The organizer of the workshop, Dr. Theodore Cole, of the University of Minnesota, explained that if the spinal cord is completely severed, there is no feeling. But if the injury is not complete, there may be body function below the level of the injury, including sexual feeling and function.

Dr. Cole says he became interested in helping wheelchair patients when he talked to a group of such men one day. "I was amazed to learn that if they had their choice between getting back their walking or their normal sexual function, they'd choose sex—it was that important to them," he said. "In the hospital we put all our effort toward the walking—we were doing nothing about sex."

Among the ways outlined by Dr. Cole for wheelchair patients to get an erection are: the partner rubbing the penis, sucking it, or putting it into her vagina and rubbing up and down on it; getting chilled; pulling at the pubic hair; putting a finger in the rectum; slapping the thigh.

DR. MICHELE'S EXERCISE FOR BETTER SEX

If you have hip or back pain during or after sexual intercourse or if you have trouble stretching your legs wide, this exercise, described by Dr. Arthur Michele in his book *Orthotherapy,* may be of help.

Stand in front of a table or bench that is about as high as your hips. Turn the foot of one leg strongly in. Stretch the other leg straight out and rest your heel on the table with your toes pointing in. Bend forward from the hip, reaching toward your outstretched foot with both hands, and bounce your torso hard, trying to reach farther toward your foot each time. Bounce 100 to 200 times, then switch to the other leg and bounce 100 to 200 times.

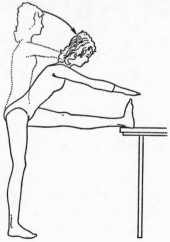

17

What to Do for Your Back during Menstruation and Pregnancy

THE PREMENSTRUAL PERIOD

Backache frequently goes along with tension, fatigue, and irritability during the premenstrual period. One theory of the cause is that muscle imbalance or weak muscles in the back and abdomen are present to begin with, and the circulatory congestion in the pelvic area at this time puts an added strain on an area that already had only minimal support. There are two avenues to correction of the problem: one to decrease the bloating and congestion in the area, and the other to increase muscle strength to better support the area.

What to do. Limit the amount of fluid you drink in the days before your menstrual period.

Eliminate salt, sugar, and carbohydrates from your diet for several days to produce water loss.

Ask your doctor about diuretic pills to rid the body of excess fluid.

If the problem is severe, have tests done to see if your body is secreting too much aldosterone hormone from the adrenal glands before your period. If so, there are medicines to counteract the problem.

Hormones sometimes help, and many women on birth-control pills say they no longer have premenstrual problems.

Have an orgasm through intercourse or masturbation. This will help pelvic congestion, sex researchers report.

106

This tip from an osteopath. Lie face down, have someone put both hands, palms crossed, in the middle of your buttocks, and gently but firmly push down on your sacrum. Or have the person sit on your buttocks and gently rock back and forth.

Nutrition aids that sometimes help to reduce premenstrual problems: vitamin A, vitamin B complex, vitamin C, calcium, vitamin E, lecithin, wheat germ, protein snacks every few hours. One doctor we talked to, who used to ignore nutrition therapy in her medical practice, says she changed her mind when she learned that blood calcium levels drop about ten days before menstruation. She found that taking calcium balanced with magnesium (sold as dolomite) eliminated her own premenstrual–menstrual backache and also reduced cramps and irritability. Further reading turned up research reports that indicated that vitamin B6 helps restore the balance of sodium and potassium and so helps prevent water being stored by the body, and that vitamin E helps regulate female sex hormones. Now she uses vitamin and mineral supplements in all her female patients with backache and other menstrual problems.

IF YOU GET BACKACHE ALONG WITH MENSTRUAL CRAMPS

What to do. Curl up with a heating pad.

Take an aspirin.

Have someone massage your back, abdomen, and legs to stimulate circulation.

Changing from physical contraceptive devices to the birth-control pill sometimes helps, or changing the kind of birth-control pills (consult your doctor).

Have an orgasm.

If your backache occurs regularly with your menstrual period, follow the same schedule of nutrition aids outlined for premenstrual backache. Have someone push down on your sacrum, as for premenstrual backache, and do the back-strengthening exercises of the Better Back Ten-Week Exercise Program.

PELVIC DISEASE

Sometimes, in pelvic infections or endometriosis (internal bleeding), adhesions and scar tissue can be produced that pull the uterus backward and add extra strain to produce backache. Other pelvic problems, such as fibroid tumors, can also produce nagging backache, especially during the menstrual period.

If your new back maintenance program does not alleviate backaches, or if your backaches are severe, discuss the problem with your family physician or your gynecologist.

WHAT TO DO FOR YOUR BACK WHEN YOU'RE PREGNANT

Backache during pregnancy may be due to increased weight, poor posture, weak muscles, or simply result from the extra strain of the big bundle in front of you, pulling your spine out of line.

The best thing to do—get physically fit before you get pregnant, and stay super-fit throughout pregnancy.

How Much Weight Should You Gain?

It is important not to gain excessive weight because the extra weight can increase back strain tremendously. Doctors used to say you should gain only ten to fourteen pounds, but present opinion is that this might have contributed to some problems in the infants. The current recommendation is to have a weight gain of twenty-four to twenty-five pounds. Keep in touch with your physician throughout pregnancy so that he may monitor your weight, nutrition, and other conditions.

Shoes

Don't wear high heels, which exaggerate the tilt of the pelvis and increase back strain. Get some safe, comfortable walking shoes with good support. They will also help prevent the falls that may occur as a result of your unaccustomed awkwardness.

How to Get Comfortable When Your Back Hurts in Pregnancy

Lie on your back with a pillow under your shoulders and head and another under your thighs just above your knees. Rotate your legs and feet outward to alleviate lower back pain. (Late in pregnancy, avoid remaining flat on your back for prolonged periods. The increased weight of the uterus may cause constriction of major blood vessels, resulting in faintness.)

Lie on your right side with a pillow or two placed diagonally under your head, breast, and shoulder. Put your right arm and leg behind you, left arm and leg in front. Allow your abdomen to rest on the bed. If necessary, place a small pillow or folded towel under the abdomen or left leg for support.

Lie flat on the floor with your heels propped on a pillow or stool. Push your back down flat. This position flattens your back, promotes good circulation to the legs, and reduces discomfort from varicose veins and leg fatigue.

When you stand, try to keep your seat tucked under, your back straight.

When you sit, keep your back straight, slide back and sit tall, with your weight evenly distributed. Your back, buttocks, and shoulders should be supported by the back of the chair. Your feet should be flat on the floor or resting on a footstool.

Do pelvic rocking to help relieve abdominal pressure and lower backache. Tighten the abdominal wall, pulling in and up, and tuck in your buttocks. This rocks the pelvis upward, flattening the lower back as you straighten the hollow there. Then slowly relax your abdomen and buttocks. Repeat 5 or 6 times, maintaining a slow, rhythmic motion. Pelvic rocking can be done when standing, sitting, lying down, or kneeling.

If you also have frequent muscle cramps, you may have a calcium deficiency. Talk to your doctor about calcium supplements.

What about a Girdle?

Many women are just as comfortable during pregnancy without a maternity girdle, but if you have persistent backache, a good maternity girdle will give extra support and help prevent back pain.

Note: If you are calmly standing at the sink or dresser and your back suddenly seems to give way and your hip kicks out with no warning when you are pregnant, not to worry. This commonly occurs because of changes in hormones near the end of pregnancy that make a major ligament relax and let go (in preparation for childbirth). Interestingly, it's the same mechanism that lets a gopher get its enlarged hips and pelvis through the little gopher hole.

HOW TO HANDLE BACKACHE DURING LABOR

Some of the backache during labor comes from muscle tension, some from extra strain and stress, and some from the fact that the baby's head has changed position and may be pushing against the lower vertebrae.

What to do. Take as much pressure as possible off the back. Adjust the pillows for maximum support.

Change your position at least every half hour.

Tip the uterus forward during contractions (pelvic rock).

Practice the relaxation and breathing exercises you learned in prenatal classes.

Have someone give you a back massage during or between contractions. A gentle back rub between contractions with greater force during the contraction is often effective.

Have your massager switch from light or hard massage to simply applying firm pressure to your back, working up and down your spine, and from one muscle to another. Between contractions put a cold compress over the lower back just up from the tailbone.

HOW TO MAKE YOUR BACK BETTER THAN EVER AFTER CHILDBIRTH

Many women have back pain after delivery because back and abdominal muscles are flabby and give little support. For getting back in shape, Dr. Gideon Panter, New York gynecologist and co-author of *Now That You've Had Your Baby*, recommends wearing a maternity girdle. During pregnancy the special pregnancy hormones caused your ligaments to relax, allowing excessive movements and extra strain on the back. Although your hormones have already changed, it takes your joints and ligaments a few weeks' time after delivery to return to a less elastic state. Wearing a girdle helps prevent all that extra movement of the joints during recovery time.

Dr. Panter also recommends the following exercises.

In the hospital and until your four- to six-week checkup—the lying-down version of the pelvic rock. Lie on your back with the knees and thighs together, knees bent at right angles, as in the Better Back Flat Back Pelvic Tilt exercise. Tuck your buttocks up and flatten your lower spine against the bed or floor. Then return and arch your back. Repeat 5 times twice a day.

After you return home, on about the tenth day—begin the pelvic eleva-tion exercise. It will strengthen both vaginal and back muscles. In the Better Back Flat Back position, raise your buttocks as in the Pelvic Raise so that your weight rests only on the soles of the feet and your shoulders, with your back straight. In this position, press your knees together and at the same time contract the abdominal and vaginal muscles as though you were trying to check a bowel movement.

At home after vaginal bleeding has stopped—the deep knee bend. It will help reestablish muscle tone in the legs as well as the back. Stand with your feet close together. At first, use a chair for sup-port. Later, as you build up strength, you can eliminate the chair. With one hand on the chair back (or resting on a wall), bend your knees until you are squatting, all the time keeping your knees pointed straight ahead. Then stand, keeping your back straight with your hips in line straight under your shoulders. Do not bend forward. Do not stick your hips out behind. Do only two or three of these at a time at first. Later you can do them 5 times, at least twice a day.

Four weeks postpartum—the pelvic rock standing. Stand with your feet slightly apart, lift your chest, pull your stomach in, pull your shoulders back and down, pull your buttocks in, and rock your pelvis forward. Rock back to the original position. Do 5 times during your regular exercise period or whenever you think of it, such as at the kitchen counter.

A good sleeping and resting position any time. This position will help get rid of the swayback you may have developed during pregnancy by helping straighten and strengthen your back. Sleep or rest while lying on your side with one or both knees drawn up high enough to make your back flexed. Lie on a firm mattress, bedboard, or even the floor. Nap often—you need the rest and relaxation time no matter how busy you are or how good you feel.

HOW TO LIFT AND CARRY AN INFANT AND SAVE YOUR BACK

Use a sling or papoose-type carrier.

Avoid one-sided carrying, which can throw your hip out of line and strain back muscles.

In lifting an infant, get as close to the child as possible, and keep it as close to your body as possible.

Bend your knees and not your back or waist, as in other save-your-back weight-lifting rules.

When you change diapers or bathe the baby, have the working level at a comfortable height so you do not have to bend over.

Put the crib mattress at as high a level as possible to avoid constant bending.

18 Helps for Menopause

Menopause usually happens around fifty but can occur later, or as early as thirty-five. Menstruation ceases, and progesterone and estrogen levels drop. It is frequently associated with osteoporosis, thus resulting in backache along with other symptoms. There is also frequently a deficiency of calcium, which causes symptoms that mimic arthritis so closely that it is often misdiagnosed. Low estrogen levels can cause backache or loss of muscle tone that may also be misdiagnosed as arthritis.

Calcium may help. The calcium level usually drops greatly when ovarian hormones decrease. Calcium is especially helpful if you have problems during the days in your cycle when you used to have premenstrual tension. Increase your calcium intake at those times. Some nutritionists claim that hot flashes, night sweats, backache, leg cramps, and irritability can sometimes disappear in a single day if you take calcium plus a little vitamin D and either vegetable or fish oil (or vitamin F) to help assimilate the calcium.

Vitamin Bs may help. B vitamins can give you peace and tranquillity to help overcome jangled nerves and resulting tensed muscles in the neck and back. Eat lots of liver, wheat germ, and brewer's yeast, or take properly balanced vitamin B complex tablets. (Don't take just one of the B vitamins; your diet should be balanced with all of them.)

Lecithin may help. It may help the body use calcium and help maintain a hormone balance.

Vitamin E may help. Because of its benefits to circulation, it is helpful for hot flashes and muscle cramps.

The estrogen controversy. Estrogen therapy has been shown to counteract weakening of bones and low back pain, to bring relief from hot flashes and sweats, and to solve the problem of vaginal tissue that often becomes dry and tender. Some doctors think it should be continued indefinitely; others use it for a short time; many, not at all. Does it cause an increased rate of cancer? Some research indicates it does; other research indicates it does not. Because evidence is still coming in and opinions changing, it is usually recommended that before starting estrogen a woman see her doctor for a checkup, that dose levels be kept as low as possible, and that women on estrogen have a twice-yearly checkup. You should not take estrogen if you have had fibroid tumors, breast cysts, or a history of cancer, or if you are obese, smoke cigarettes, have high blood pressure, or high levels of cholesterol or triglycerides.

Note: Many women find that if they take 1 to 5 mg. of folic acid, symptoms of backaches and vaginal dryness disappear so they no longer need to take estrogen. Folic acid has also been reported to increase sexual desire. In the United States a prescription is needed for these amounts, but not in Canada.

Caution: If menstrual bleeding stops for many months, then starts again, if you have spotting between periods, or if bleeding becomes especially heavy, call your doctor immediately.

19 What You Should Know about Sports and Your Back

It isn't just orthopedic specialists and neurosurgeons who know a lot about backs. Coaches and physicians to the major sports teams frequently deal with back problems. Often they have some unique insights or special techniques that can be helpful to the average person with a back problem, or for that matter to anyone who wants to help protect themselves or their children from back problems. I gathered material from these experts in the field about every major sport and how it might relate to your back.

THE THREE SPORTS MOST OFTEN RECOMMENDED BY BACK EXPERTS TO BUILD YOUR BACK

Walking—Increase the distance and briskness with time.

Jogging—Be sure not to run with a swayback, work up gradually, and run on a soft surface with good shoes.

Swimming—The backstroke is especially good.

(See the following pages for more details on the best ways to use these sports to build your back.)

These sports will also give you the highest fitness benefit for your heart, lungs, and entire body.

Sports for building up back, heart, and lungs should be done at least three times a week for maximum benefit.

NINE BASIC RULES FOR ANY SPORT
IF YOU HAVE A WEAK BACK

Get your doctor's approval before starting.

Begin gradually and build up time and endurance in gradual stages.

If any particular sport or movement produces pain, avoid it.

Spend a few minutes walking or doing warm-up exercises appropriate to the sport before each strenuous session.

Avoid sudden, awkward jarring moves. A quick shift off balance can throw even a healthy back askew.

Choose a sport that releases tension, not adds to it.

Don't do it with a swayback; keep your back straight.

If you are a weekender only, be sure to do vigorous walking or other exercising during the week to avoid being out of shape, most hazardous to your back.

Keep up the Better Back Program conditioning exercises to make your back stronger and less vulnerable to injury.

HAZARDOUS SPORTS IF YOU HAVE A BAD BACK

You should avoid sports that involve rough physical contact, where there is dangerous physical stress to your back, where there is twisting or arching, or where there is danger of sudden impact or jarring. Thus the following sports are contraindicated for anyone with a bad back: basketball, board diving, bowling, football, handball, high-jumping, hurdles, ice hockey, pole vaulting, sledding and tobogganing, snowmobiling, soccer, trampoline, volleyball, weight-lifting, and wrestling.

Sports that can be good or bad, depending on whether you are skilled and whether you can keep your back straight when participating instead of arched, include the following: golf, horseback riding, ice skating, jogging and running, karate, jujitsu, skiing, tennis. For any of these sports, obtain professional instruction if you have a bad back to be sure that you are using the proper nonstressing techniques. If you have strengthened your back through the Better Back Program exercises and if you play moderately within your ability, these sports should not give you trouble. If you want to engage in these sports, check with your doctor first and begin cautiously, building up endurance.

EXPERTS' TIPS ON SPECIFIC SPORTS

Jogging

Dangers. Some experts estimate that half of all runners and joggers will experience some kind of painful injury to the feet, legs, knees, or back.

Is it good for your back? If you have a healthy back, jogging and running are excellent conditioners. If you have a back problem, there could be trouble if you do not have proper form, coordination, training, and skill. Check with your doctor first and get proper guidance.

What experts recommend. Get off on the right foot by getting into condition first, says Duke University track coach Al Buehler, who was a manager of the U.S. track team at the Munich Olympics. He says if you are thirty-five or over, you should see a physician before beginning a running program, and all new runners should approach the sport "slowly and easily." A back-saver: run only on soft surfaces like park fields and athletic trails rather than concrete and asphalt, which are punishing to bones and muscles, including those of the back. Type of running shoe? Buehler recommends the training flat with uppers of nylon and suede and soles of thick rubber with arch support. Once you find a comfortable shoe that doesn't produce injuries, stick to it, he says, since many running injuries occur when runners switch from one brand of shoe to another. And when you get a new pair of shoes, he says, start breaking them in before the old ones fall apart so the body will adapt to the new shoes.

Advice from Jesse Owens, immortal Olympic track star: relax. "I had a coach who taught me how to relax when moving. It not only made me run faster but made me look like what I was doing was easy," he says. "I remember my coach once saying to me, 'Jesse, did you ever see a horse run? He doesn't waste energy gritting his teeth or tensing his muscles in determined looks. He just runs for the pure joy of running, with his whole body working together.'"

Track coach William J. Bowerman and heart specialist Dr. W. E. Harris, authors of *Jogging,* advise joggers to keep the back as straight as is naturally comfortable. "Keep your head up, neither forward nor back of the body line," they say. "Your buttocks should be tucked in." They warn not to imitate the military posture of throwing back the shoulders and sticking out the chest. "If you do, you're likely to get a muscle ache between the shoulder blades and some discomfort in the lower back. And you will use a lot of energy by unnecessarily contracting a whole series of back muscles." If you develop mild soreness, they suggest you continue your schedule of jogging. If soreness is severe, cut down to walking on schedule and build back up gradually to regular jogging. For low back pain, they recommend the wall stand (Better Back Exercise 4) and the Flat Back Pelvic Tilt (Exercise 3).

Other advice. Some doctors said that running, because it is a smoother gliding motion, is easier on the spine than the more up-and-down motion of jogging. Running on sand is extremely strenuous. If you do it, run on the beach where the water comes in and the sand is firmer; it places less stress on the back.

Run in an upright position; don't lean. Don't run with a swayback. Keep your back as straight as you can and still remain comfortable. Don't look at your feet.

Breathe deeply with your mouth open. Do not hold your breath.

If you become unusually tired or uncomfortable, slow down, walk, or stop.

Do not wear rubberized or plastic clothing, which can cause the body temperature to rise to dangerous levels.

Wear thick-soled shoes and soft, well-fitting socks. Both will help cushion jarring to the spine.

Don't jog during the first hour after eating, or during the middle of a hot humid day.

Don't jog or run downhill; it puts excessive strain on the knees and back. Walk when you come to a downhill slope.

Tennis

Dangers. Straining a muscle; injuring the knees, hips, or back by pounding on a hard court.

Is it good for your back? Some doctors say tennis is not good for an ailing back; some doctors who have had back trouble themselves say it is the only thing that cured their pain because it built up the back muscles and improved their general condition. Check with your doctor.

What experts recommend. Take lessons from a pro; poor

strokes, such as hitting the ball too late, cause more tennis injuries than anything else. Get in condition before you start playing; when you do start, build up the intensity and time of your playing gradually. Warm up with some limbering exercises before you go on the court. For the first few days, take a hot shower or hot tub soak after the workout to prevent later stiffness and discomfort. If you are a weekend player, keep in condition between games. If you have a bad back, avoid arching your back in hard serves or overhead smashes, and don't hit the ball if you are in an awkward position.

What are the physical requirements for a good tennis player? Strength and stamina, says Billie Jean King. "For a powerful serve and overhead he or she must have a solid stomach and a strong back." She recommends running and rope skipping to build up endurance, but *after* a game or on rainy days, not before a game, because you need all the strength and concentration for the game itself. One of her favorite abdominal and back strengthening exercises is the kangaroo hop. "From a standing position, jump straight up in the air as high as you can," she explains, "and, while keeping your back straight, clasp your knees to your chest with your arms. If you can work up to fifty of these quickly and without stopping (thirty for women), consider yourself in superb shape."

What to do if your back starts to bother you? Dieter Eber, a Wimbledon winner and German star of the senior tennis division, says to stay off hard-surface courts and play only on clay. If he has problems, he gets a vitamin B$_{12}$ shot and takes supplementary B vitamins. Christoph Thomas-Morr, German national doubles champion, is often bothered by neck and back discomfort. "Before a tournament I always take vitamin B complex and vitamin C tablets," he says. "And if I have any problems I do back-strengthening exercises and hang from an overhead bar I have installed in my basement." His doctor, Dr. Kurt Becker, who is also a physician to the German Olympic team, has Thomas-Morr do the backstroke when he swims.

Well-known surgeon Dr. William Nolen, author of several medical books and columnist for *McCalls* magazine, says that he tells his back patients to lose weight to reduce strain on the back and to practice regular graduated exercises for strengthening back muscles. However, when he suffers backache himself, he says he takes aspirin, uses a heating pad, swears when he tries to

put on his pants, and as soon as the acute attack is over, he goes
back to tennis or other sports.

Walking and Hiking

Dangers. Back strain from carrying too heavy a load when
hiking; falling on rugged terrain.

Is it good for your back? Walking is very good, but not
backpacking if you have a bad back, most doctors said.

What experts recommend. Wear comfortable shoes when you
walk or hike. For most benefit to your body, walk briskly. Extend
the time and distance until you are walking at least half an hour a
day if you are not engaging in other exercise.

Watch out for "rucksack palsy" from hiking with a heavy load
on your back. It used to be a common complaint of marching
soldiers. The symptoms include pain, numbness, and weakness in
the back, shoulders, and arms because of pressure of the
backpack on nerves and blood vessels. Use a backpack with metal
supports to distribute the load onto hips and thick foam-rubber
cushioning under the shoulder straps. There should be as little
pressure on the shoulders as possible, since this tends to increase
lordosis. At the first sign of discomfort, remove and lighten pack.
If you have back trouble, don't carry a backpack at all.

Swimming

Dangers. Injury or back strain from jumping or diving.

Is it good for your back? One of the best exercises you can do
for both the healthy back and the back that needs help is swimming, but you need to really swim, not just paddle and splash
around. Swimming is especially good for those with stiff muscles
because the buoyancy of the water allows freer action. In fact,
many physical therapists specifically give exercise treatment in
water to increase and maintain mobility of the joints and
strengthen muscles. A person immersed up to the neck in water
experiences a relaxing loss of 90 percent of his weight.

What experts recommend. The backstroke is the best back
strengthener. The crawl and sidestroke are also good if you can
keep your back from arching as you do them. (If you tilt your chin

sideways, not up, this will help avoid arching of the back.) The breast or butterfly stroke should be avoided because it develops the wrong muscles and arches the back. Holding on the side of the pool and kicking is a good hip exercise (keep the back straight). If you use a kickboard, put it under your chest for support so your back is not arched. Work up to swimming distances gradually. If you have a bad back, don't dive off the board.

Many doctors recommended swimming to strengthen the back and spine after injury. A typical example—Monika Tilley, a fashion designer who suffered a near-fatal back injury while water-skiing and was completely immobilized. She was able to walk again after four weeks of a total relaxation treatment program plus a week of intensive swimming in the Cayman Islands, and still does back-stretching exercises and swims regularly to keep her back muscles toned up.

Micki King, Olympic swimming and diving champion and fitness coordinator for the first women cadets entering the U.S. Air Force Academy, stresses the need for warm-up exercises before swimming, diving, or other sports, keeping the movements rhythmic, not bouncing. For stretching the lower back, she uses the Single Knee Raise (Exercise 5).

Joanne P. Levy, physical therapist and author of *Ouch! My Back Is Killing Me!*, says that during an attack of back pain one should avoid swimming in water below 70 degrees and should take a hot shower after swimming to avoid getting chilled.

As a first exercise to do in the water for back pain (after a period of bed rest), Levy recommends walking in water. Again be sure to keep the arch out of your back as you walk.

Snorkeling is okay whether you have a bad back or not; for skin diving you will have to test for yourself to see if jackknifing to go down puts too much strain on your back.

Scuba diving is permissible since the tanks are at neutral buoyancy in the water, but do not walk around on land with the heavy tanks strapped to your back.

Golf

Dangers. Improper twisting and straining.

Is it good for your back? Opinions differ. Experts stressed, however, that the person with a bad back who cannot play without getting tense should avoid the game. If relaxed, the walking involved can be good for the back. Check with your doctor.

What experts recommend. Do not lean backward at the completion of the swing in an attempt to watch the ball. Concentrate on relaxed playing and on keeping the body in complete alignment and balance. Limit the hours you play until you have tested the effect of the game on your back.

Also watch how you bend over, says Dr. Marilyn Moffat, of New York University. "Most people," she says, "tend to hang over at a right angle when placing or retrieving the golf ball. Squatting or bending at the hips and knees rather than the waist, helps to alleviate stress on the spine."

Bicycling

Dangers. Falling or overdoing.

Is it good for your back? Yes, if you maintain good posture.

What experts recommend. Don't ride with a backpack. Choose a bicycle with handlebars that help you keep your back straight instead of hunched over or with lordosis. Wear chain guards to avoid getting slacks caught in the chains, sending you sailing over the handlebars onto your head, or injuring your spine.

Dr. Paul Dudley White, famed heart specialist and a doctor to presidents, was famous for riding a bicycle around Washington when he was in his seventies. He recommended bike riding to many back patients with good results.

Skiing

Dangers. Falling or twisting the back or hitting trees or hidden rocks.

Is it good for your back? Skiing is an excellent exercise for the entire body. But, except for cross-country, if you have a bad back the dangers of twisting and falling from skiing are too great to risk the strain on the back.

What experts recommend. See that your skis and boots are in good condition. Adjust your release bindings tighter for powdery snow, looser for deep-packed snow. Use releases that permit immediate sideways release in leg-twisting falls. Get professional instruction. Stick to bunny slopes until the pro says you're ready for bigger things. Get off the runs before you're tired. (More accidents occur in late afternoon than any other time because of skier fatigue.) Stay off slopes marked unsafe.

Do conditioning exercises before the season starts and between ski trips, especially those meant to strengthen the torso and the legs. Swimming, cycling, jumping rope, jogging, walking, and stair climbing are good conditioning activities. Do halfway knee bends, stopping as if you were sitting in midair and holding the position as long as you can. Walk about on your toes (keep your back straight), do the half sit-ups and leg raises outlined in the Better Back Exercise Program.

Back expert Dr. Hans Kraus stresses that people in poor condition run a much greater risk of injury than others. He deplores the poor condition of persons on the ski slopes today, and tells the story of a friend who runs a ski school near New York who said she had to refuse lessons to many beginners because they did not have enough strength to get up once they had fallen to the ground. "I found it hard to believe," says Kraus, "but on my next visit to that resort I actually saw people who were completely unable to get up off the snow, even though they were in the correct position to get up. This was even true of a number of children."

Dr. Richard M. Suinn, chairman of the department of psychology at Colorado State University and psychologist consultant to the U.S. Olympic ski team, recommends relaxation techniques plus mental imagery to increase performance and thus reduce mishaps. For several sessions he has the U.S. skiers learn progressive relaxation. Later they can become relaxed physically and mentally in seconds to counteract the pressure of competition. In mental imagery the skiers practice skiing techniques simply by imagining moment-by-moment a downhill race with jumps, rough sections, fast sections, right to the skidding stop past the finish line. Something similar to this technique was reported used by three-time winner of Olympic gold medals Jean-Claude Killy. He was recovering from an injury at the time and couldn't practice, so his only preparation for one race was to ski it mentally. The race turned out to be one of his best.

Basketball

Dangers. Surprisingly, recent statistics show that basketball is one of the most dangerous team sports. There were more injuries connected with it than with either baseball or football.

Is it good for your back? For the person with a healthy back, there is no problem. For the person with a bad back, there are too many twistings, turnings, and sudden movements.

What experts recommend. Get into prime condition before playing, concentrating especially on leg-strengthening exercises to help protect knees and ankles from being sprained or dislocated from the sudden wrenches of twisting and turning in the game. Do not go back to the game too soon after an injury; get approval from your doctor first. Baskets should always be positioned to leave ample room behind them so players are not in danger of colliding with a wall or into spectators sitting too close.

Football

Dangers. The Department of Health, Education and Welfare estimates as many as a million injuries annually. And football injuries can be more serious than those suffered in other sports. The chances for permanent injury are overwhelming, says NYU Dr. Hans Kraus. Injuries may include shock to the spine that causes problems immediately or later in life or can be as serious as quadriplegia or death. Biggest danger: head impact in blocking and tackling, striking the head or faceguard with the knee, clotheslining, sharp bending of the neck.

Is it good for your back? Not at any age or any time. Football is an extremely dangerous sport for the head, neck, and spine. At one university, freshmen football players were X-rayed and 32 percent were found to have fractures, disk problems, and limited motion just from playing in high school football, all disabilities of which they were unaware. The Arthritis Foundation says 50 to 80 percent of high school and college football players are eventually injured and many, because of the injuries, will have serious painful arthritis later in life. Ex-football players are notorious for having back problems later in life as a result of minor daily injuries from the game.

Dr. Joseph S. Torg, professor of orthopedic surgery at the

University of Pennsylvania School of Medicine, who has observed many fatalities and cases of paralysis from the game, says the true statistics on football injuries are only now becoming completely known. He calls it "a significant national health problem," and says pinching and stretching injuries to the spine usually happen to several members of a team at any game, causing them to have a shocklike sensation, temporary paralysis, and temporary loss of sensation. Torg reports such cases as a seventeen-year-old high school boy who collided with a spring-loaded blocking dummy and died two days later. Another boy was participating in a sandlot pickup game. He tried to head-butt a tackler and dislocated the vertebrae in his neck. He remains a quadriplegic, unable to walk, feed himself, or have bowel or bladder control. He was fifteen!

It happens in pro football too. Take the Stingley family of football players. Harold Stingley, a running back with the Brown Bombers, broke his neck playing. His son Darryl, the New England Patriots' star receiver, suffered a broken neck in a game with the Oakland Raiders. Darryl's older brother Wayne suffered a traumatic blow to the spine.

Back problems are particularly common in linemen, defensive ends, guards, tackles, and centers, according to Dr. Roger J. Ferguson, orthopedic surgeon at the University of Pittsburgh. He found that during a recent year *50 percent* of linemen studied at one university sought medical attention for low back pain. The stance that a lineman takes makes him particularly susceptible to injury, Dr. Ferguson says. "He drives forward and upward as he collides with his fellow players and tries to push them backward." Most of the collision force is absorbed at the vertebral joints, he says, often causing repeated fractures, and the residual damage can cause back problems for life.

What experts recommend. Don't play, or if you do, be in top physical condition. Any person, even children, should have a thorough physical examination before participating in football of *any* kind. Other things to insist on: strong supervised preseason and throughout-the-season conditioning with emphasis on strengthening of the neck; wearing proper equipment, including well-fitted helmet; rigidly observed safety rules; avoidance of using the head and helmet to spear or butt an opposing player; avoidance of amphetamine pep pills that encourage players to take unnecessary risks; outlawing of self-propelled blocking and tackling dummies.

What if a player is injured? Before he ever returns to competition, he should undergo a strenuous remedial program, says the American Medical Association. It should include a strengthening program for the neck, shoulders, and upper back; checking protective equipment to make sure it is in good condition, fits properly, and is worn correctly; evaluation of playing techniques; and a final examination by the team physician.

Baseball

Dangers. Injury from sliding into a base, getting hit by a ball or bat.

Is it good for your back? For the person with a strong back, baseball is permissible. For the person with a weak back, there is too much twisting and turning, too many sudden jerky movements.

What experts recommend. Never fling the bat away after hitting the ball—it becomes a dangerous weapon; just drop it. Only slide into base feet first; head-first slides can cause serious injury to the head and spine. Keep your eye on the ball at all times or you may get beaned.

Special advice for children. To prevent "Little League elbow," Dr. Kenneth DeHaven, of Cleveland Clinic, offers the following advice. Have any young pitcher do easy conditioning warm-up pitches before going into the game; limit young pitchers to a maximum of two innings of pitching per game, and ban the use of a curve ball or other trick pitches. Children's arms and shoulders are not ready for that kind of stress, and serious damage can be done to developing muscles, bones, and joint connections. If a child reports soreness, strain, or an inability to fully extend the arm after pitching, insist he stop playing and have the arm evaluated by a physician. Continued throwing can cause severe problems, including fractures, arthritis, and permanent loss of elbow extension, Dr. DeHaven warns.

Dancing

Dangers. Doing the twist, complicated ballet steps, or other stressful dances can strain your back.

Is it good for your back? Yes, just avoid the twist, the duck walk, splits, and other fancy maneuvers. Done properly, dancing can help extend the spine, improve posture, and increase coordination. And it helps use up calories and keeps you trim. Bob Hope has an extra-long cord on his telephone and says he does old vaudeville tap dance routines while talking on the phone.

What experts recommend. Jacki Sorensen, head of the Aerobic Dancing Studio, in Northridge, California, says not to dance on hard surfaces such as concrete, to keep knees loose and relaxed while dancing, to keep the back straight and in proper alignment, and to move mainly on the front half of your feet or even flat-footed, but not high on your toes. The proper body alignment when dancing, she says, is to pull the stomach in and up, tuck the seat under, the shoulders back and down, and to stand tall and relaxed. If your abdominal muscles hang loose when you dance, she warns, you could strain lower back muscles.

Horseback Riding

Dangers. Being thrown off, stepped or rolled on, kicked by a flailing hoof, slashed by rope burns, bitten, or hit by low-hanging tree limbs.

What experts recommend. Wear a helmet. Check saddle, stirrups, and bridle carefully and frequently. Stay alert to the horse and to overhanging tree limbs. Ride with your back straight, not with an exaggerated curve in it.

Is it good for your back? If you have a bad back, you should check with your doctor and also test the effect for yourself since different people with different conditions seem to react in different ways. Many doctors felt riding was especially bad for low-back pain sufferers and those with disk problems.

If you have a healthy back, riding can be good exercise. In fact, horseman Dr. William Barclay points out in the *Journal of the American Medical Association,* of which he is an editor, that the risk of injury is low for the expert horseman, and a person can participate in equestrian activities even at an advanced age. "As a matter of personal observation, a day's ride on my hunter not only refreshes my spirits," he says, "but also seems to relieve the chronic backache that is aggravated by long hours of sitting at the editor's desk."

Gymnastics

Dangers. Twisting the back, overextending or overflexing the spine, falling on the spine, fractures of the spine.

Is it good for your back? No. Dr. Douglas Jackson, orthopedic surgeon of the University of California at Irvine, reported at a recent meeting of the American College of Sports Medicine that fatigue fracture and slippage of the vertebrae occur 400 percent more often in gymnasts than in the general population. There is also a high incidence of spine defects in persons participating in karate, hurdling, pole-vaulting, and high jumping, he said. In one group of 100 girls in year-round gymnastic training, Dr. Jackson found 11 had spine damage, and 19 others had low back pain severe enough to curtail their workouts. In fact, he says, some of the world's top competitors in gymnastics have had to be immobilized in hospitals from time to time for back problems.

What experts recommend. Be particularly wary of back and front walkovers, dismounting, vaulting, and flipping. If you have back pain or are unable to do your routines, see a doctor immediately.

Avoid trampolines. In fact, the American Academy of Pediatrics has officially advised that trampolines should be banned from schools and competition. My dear friend the late Dr. Harvey Kravitz, who was a member of the Academy committee making the recommendation, said hundreds of serious spine injuries have occurred on trampolines in the last decade. In fact, a national survey of sports in high schools and colleges showed that spinal cord injuries with permanent paralysis resulted more often from trampolines than from any other gymnastic activity. (Only football caused more.)

Somersaulting is especially dangerous whether in gymnastics, football, or track, since it can cause a broken neck or back. Such grandstand tricks as New Zealander trackman John Delamere's forward somersault at the beginning of his long jump is extremely dangerous to the spine, doctors say. They also are worried that since high jumper Dick Fosbury used a backward flop over the high-jump bar in the Olympics other young athletes will try the somersaults and flops with the danger of spine injuries and paralysis.

PHYSICIANS LOOK AT CHILDREN AND SPORTS

In 1972, *Medical World News,* a physicians' magazine, ran a report by British radiologist Dr. Ronald O. Murray that 24 percent of boys in British prep schools that stressed athletics, had hip problems, especially of the head of the hip bones. The condition often occurs in children who are overweight and out of condition when they get into sports, doctors say.

The study goes along with others that have shown how much out of condition today's children often are. In fact, according to the President's Council on Physical Fitness and Sports, one out of every six children in the United States is so weak, uncoordinated, or generally inept that he or she cannot pass the simple standards of physical fitness outlined by the Council. The average child today spends less than 1 percent of his time in physical activity and 10 percent watching TV, the Council says.

And it is being out of condition that is the major cause of the back and other injuries that occur to children when they participate in sports.

How to Help Your Child from Being Injured in Sports

What you do for your child now can not only help protect him from injury in childhood sports, but can help him or her develop and keep a strong back that will affect his or her life in later years.

Jets' physician Dr. James A. Nicholas urges exercise programs to build muscle strength and general fitness, both on an individual basis and in schools.

The President's Council on Physical Fitness and the American Medical Association have called for screening of all schoolchildren to find those who are undeveloped or in need of special exercise and treatment for muscle and bone disorders. (Although this is not being done on a national scale, the tests in this book will help you check your own child and make some determinations about what his or her exercise program should be, in consultation with your pediatrician.)

Dr. William F. Collins, professor of surgery and chief of neurosurgery at Yale University School of Medicine, believes children should be encouraged to take up sports they can enjoy all their lives, like tennis and swimming, rather than team sports. He cites members of the Scandinavian royal families who continue to play tennis to age seventy and eighty as examples to follow. "You can tell by the way these men and women walk that they have few back problems."

Avoid intense competition for your child in any sport, says Dr. Hans Kraus, especially if it makes the child push himself beyond his limits. He will be playing under tension before the game even begins, laying himself open to injury.

Help your child get good muscle function with exercises to improve coordination and strength and avoid the poor muscle function that creates awkwardness and clumsiness at sports and leads to injury.

Give him or her professional instruction when possible so self-confidence and proper skills are developed right from the beginning.

Every doctor questioned said: Don't push the child. Don't goad him or her beyond their abilities, or put so much stress on winning.

Let your child have fun without any goals. You want your child to enjoy physical activity so he doesn't grow up to be a sedentary, overweight, flabby adult with all of the added health risks that those conditions entail.

Four Conditions That May Be Responsible for Back Pain in Young Athletes

Even when back pain seems obviously caused by an injury during athletics, there can be an underlying back problem that produced both the pain and the injury that occurred, doctors told me, so anyone sustaining a back injury in sports should be thoroughly examined for underlying problems.

Dr. John H. McMaster, orthopedic surgeon and director of sports medicine at the University of Pittsburgh, outlined the following five major causes for such back pain in a report at an American Medical Association Conference on the Medical Aspects of Sports.

Curvature of the spine. Called scoliosis by physicians, this condition is common in adolescents. Exercises and braces can usually correct the condition without surgery. (See Chapter 32, Special Problems of Children, for more details.)

Scheuermann's disease. This disease, also called round-back or kyphosis, was described by a Dr. Scheuermann in 1921. The peak incidence occurs in boys and girls between the ages of thirteen and seventeen. Patients usually have a prominent protruding abdomen as well and are often simply thought to have poor posture. It can be diagnosed by the wedge shapes of the vertebrae at X-ray.

Spondylolysis and Spondylolisthesis. These two conditions are similar and usually involve fracture of part of a vertebra because of physical stress. Sometimes rest is all that is needed; in more severe cases or in children whose bones have not matured, surgery is often necessary. In some cases, one physician said, the condition may produce no symptoms in the well-conditioned athlete, but will appear later if that athlete becomes an overweight, flabby businessman.

Herniated disk. Although this condition is more likely to occur in adults, it can be seen in children, especially those at about age twelve who are undergoing rapid skeletal growth. Diagnostic signs include muscle spasm and limitation of motion of the spine, and pain which occurs in the straight-leg-raising test.

WOMEN AND SPORTS

Today more girls than ever are becoming involved in athletics. (If you think your school is not giving equal opportunities to girls in athletics, check to see who their Title IX coordinator is, or contact SPRINT, a national information center on sex equality in sports that is based in Washington, D.C.)

Is the new trend safe for developing girls? Injury rates for girls in interscholastic sports are no greater than those for boys in the same games, says a report in the *Journal of the American Medical Association.* Dr. James G. Garrick, director of the St. Francis Center for Sports Medicine in San Francisco, and Ralph Requa, research director for the Margaret Goldwater Foundation for Research and Education, Sun City, Arizona, said there were no differences in rates of injuries to the back or other parts of the body in badminton, basketball, cross-country, gymnastics, softball, swimming, tennis, track and field, or volleyball. Girls in the study did not participate in football or wrestling.

Dr. Joan Ullyot, a physiologist at San Francisco's Institute of Health Research, says in fact that the evidence suggests that

women are tougher than men in many ways. A world-class
marathoner herself, she says women often outrun men in ultra-
long marathon races of fifty miles.

What about female organs? "A man's scrotum is much more
vulnerable than a woman's ovaries," says Dr. John Marshall, director of sports medicine at Manhattan's Hospital for Special
Surgery and consultant to Billie Jean King. A woman's breasts
also are not easily damaged, he says.

A girl's training can be just as vigorous as a boy's, says Dr.
Barbara Drinkwater, physiologist at the University of California
Institute of Environmental Stress. She found that girls test just the
same as boys in heart-lung endurance. And women can increase
their strength tremendously with training. Dr. Jack Wilmore,
president of the American College of Sports Medicine, and Dr.
C. Harmon Brown found women could increase their strength by
more than 50 percent and still not increase their muscle bulk so
they looked like Lady Tarzans. They found women's legs were
usually as strong as men's in the same condition, but that men's
arms generally were twice as strong because their arms are longer
and their shoulders broader.

20 What Diet, Vitamins, and Minerals Can Do for Your Back

Our national diet is so poor that the recent United States Senate Select Committee on Nutrition and Human Needs reported it was linked to at least six of the ten leading causes of death—heart disease, cancer, strokes, diabetes, hardening of the arteries, and cirrhosis of the liver. Poor diet can affect your back, too.

Many of the doctors we talked to cited a change in diet as a way to make your back stronger.

Diet can help in two ways. First, it can provide vitamins and minerals needed to make bones strong, to keep them from getting soft or brittle. Bone is not an inert material. It is alive and always changing, constantly building up and breaking down its components. It vitally needs certain things in the diet. Second, a proper diet can help you lose weight if you are obese—one of the biggest causes of backache.

You may be careful not to lift heavy things, but if you are overweight you lift a heavy weight every day, constantly straining your back. If you also have a potbelly, with weak abdominal muscles, that strains the back even more, increasing the curve of the back and putting a constant forward pull on struggling back muscles.

So getting rid of excess weight and staying slim for life is one of the most important things you can do to get rid of back pain, if you already have it, or to protect your back from future trouble. In fact, at one recent meeting of an orthopedic society the three

133

most important treatments cited for curing low back pain were exercising, improving posture, and maintaining proper weight. More than 95 percent of 749 patients treated with that combination over a fifteen-month period were relieved of pain. Sometimes, doctors told us, a loss of only ten pounds can bring relief.

THE BETTER-BACK DIET

The diet we give you here is designed both to help you overcome deficiencies in the vitamins and minerals that have been shown to be most related to preventing and overcoming back problems and to help you stay slim and so reduce strain on your back.

1. Eliminate sugar completely. Read labels when you buy so you avoid baked, canned, or frozen foods or drinks with hidden sugar.

2. Eliminate refined carbohydrates, such as white bread, white rice, macaroni, spaghetti, cakes, or cookies. Eat whole grains instead.

3. Eliminate processed, imitation, and synthetic foods as much as possible. Eat fresh foods instead.

4. Limit fats and oils to moderate amounts. (Don't eliminate them completely; you need adequate amounts for hormones, smooth skin, natural lubrication.)

5. Limit your intake of coffee, tea, and cola drinks to moderate amounts, especially if you tend to be tense, anxious, or irritable from caffeine or have insomnia. But do drink plenty of liquids.

6. Limit alcohol to moderate amounts.

7. Eat as wide a variety as you can of whole grain foods, fruits, salads, vegetables, and adequate amounts of fish, poultry, eggs, meats, or cheese.

8. Take a vitamin-mineral supplement. Consult with a doctor well versed in nutrition to be sure you are getting proper amounts of vitamins and minerals, particularly those cited as most frequently missing in today's diet, and find out whether you should be taking any more or less of certain vitamins or minerals.

Note: Tell your doctor your plans to change to this diet. Check to see if you have any chronic conditions that would be affected by the diet or if you are taking any medications that would have to be changed on such a diet.

Some Ways to Make the Diet Easy for Yourself

Don't keep candy, cookies, cakes, pies, and sugared drinks in the house. Don't worry if your children eat things at weird times, as long as they eat *good* things. And don't worry if young children drink a lot of water. They need extra fluids. Let them eat between meals if they wish, but make the snacks nutritious. Children feel hungry more often than adults, but cannot eat as much at one sitting.

Set up a self-service snack center . . . one or two shelves in the refrigerator, where everyone knows to reach, and on the counter next to the refrigerator; keep both filled with nutritious foods. Allowable treats: milk, fruit juices, cottage cheese, yogurt, cheeses, leftover meats, melon slices, carrot and celery sticks, cauliflower buds, radishes, cabbage leaves, green peppers, tomatoes, tangerines, apples, oranges, grapefruits, bananas, dried apricots, dates, figs, prunes, whole wheat crackers or whole grain bread. In the freezer you might have individual containers of frozen yogurt.

Fix as wide a variety of food as possible, since different foods contain different nutrients.

Keep vitamin and mineral supplements on the kitchen counter at all times so it's easy to grab your daily supply at meal times.

Read labels and choose foods selectively. (Ingredients are listed in order of their relative quantity in a food.)

Visit a health food store. See if there is anything there that appeals to you: papaya juice, sunflower seeds.

Don't overcook things. Eat food garden-fresh and still crispy, gourmet style.

Cook with as little water as possible. Use leftover cooking water for soups or stews; use leftover vegetables like asparagus, beans, beets, and peas in salads the next day instead of cooking them again and causing more nutrient loss.

Keep track of your back symptoms and whether they change as you lose weight.

Go Ahead and Nibble

On this diet it's okay to nibble even if you are trying to lose weight. Research with animals shows that animals fed many times a day gain less weight than those fed the same total of food in only three meals. Many people find it very helpful to eat a protein snack of cheese, fowl, fish, beans, or nuts every three hours, or to take fructose tablets (from your pharmacist or health food store) for long-lasting energy. Just make sure your snacks are not weight-producing sweets and starches. Or try eating five little meals a day instead of three large ones.

FINDING OUT WHAT VITAMINS AND MINERALS YOU NEED

Many physicians believe the current recommendations of daily requirement of vitamins and minerals that are given by the government are much lower than they should be. They feel that for optimum health and elimination of many symptoms plaguing our everyday lives, much higher doses of vitamins and minerals are necessary—super-nutrition. Other physicians do not agree and, in fact, say that our diets today are perfectly okay.

I have talked to hundreds of patients who, after trying a no-sugar, no-refined starches diet, plus high amounts of vitamins and minerals and exercise, found their backaches and other problems disappeared. But the most convincing evidence was talking to doctors who once felt that vitamins and minerals were a waste of time and money until they were open-minded enough to test them on their patients and saw for themselves how the patients' problems were improved.

One doctor, for example, uses large doses of vitamin C for patients with back problems, finding it often relieves pain and increases mobility significantly. He also used it to get relief from his own back pain, which had bothered him for some ten years. Vitamin C is important, he says, because it is essential to the formation of connective tissue in bones, cartilage, and ligaments.

Different doctors have such widely differing opinions on vitamin needs that it is difficult for a patient to know how to make a decision that is best. One way to get an objective answer is by an individualized laboratory test. Computer analysis of your daily diet and hair analysis offer the most accurate methods of telling what vitamins and minerals you are deficient in. For the diet analysis, you fill out a detailed questionnaire about foods you usually eat. For the hair analysis, you put a small sample of your hair, cut close to the scalp, in an envelope and send it to a laboratory which analyzes it by computer techniques to determine what you have too much or too little of that can be causing symptoms. Your doctor can order a hair analysis as well as a diet analysis for you from Bio-Medical Data, Inc., P.O. Box 6118, Chicago, Illinois 60680. They will send back a report on your body levels of fifteen minerals plus recommendations for any restructuring of your diet that may be needed.

If the hair or diet analysis indicates you have deficiencies, or if you have other reasons for believing you have deficiencies, ask your doctor to help you work out a proper balance of supplements. If your regular doctor does not wish to do this, you can contact any of the following organizations for the name of a local specialist in the field. Be sure to state the nature of your problem so the most appropriate referral will be given to you. And remember to enclose a stamped, self-addressed envelope with your inquiry.

International Academy of Metabology, 2236 Suree Ellen Lane, Altadena, California 91001.

International College of Applied Nutrition, Box 386, La Habra, California 90631.

International Academy of Preventative Medicine, 871 Frostwood Drive, Houston, Texas 77024.

Huxley Institute for Biosocial Research, 1114 First Avenue, New York, New York 10021.

DIET AND HEALING OF FRACTURES

We heard many stories from doctors and patients alike of better healing resulting from large amounts of vitamins and minerals. One case concerned a seventy-nine-year-old man with a shoulder so badly shattered in so many little pieces that the surgeon said it was impossible for him to repair it by surgery. After several weeks of conventional therapy the bone had still not begun to heal. However, it did begin healing when bone meal, supplements of calcium, magnesium, zinc, and vitamins D and C were added to his diet in large amounts. X-rays showed that complete function has now returned and the patient can pursue a normal life.

Also see Chapter 33, When Surgery Is Necessary.

THE STORY OF CALCIUM

Calcium may be the single most important ingredient in a diet for your back. It is absolutely essential for strong bones. Without it, your bones slowly soften and weaken, often fracturing from the slightest blow because they are so brittle.

In fact, a deficiency in calcium is one of the biggest factors in causing osteoporosis, the bone weakening that often happens with aging.

About one in four women and one in eight men has the bone deterioration of osteoporosis. The bone weakness causes the fractures that occur so often in older people after minor falls, as well as "dowager's hump," loss of height, and back pain. In fact, often when many people are thought to fall down and break their hip, their hip actually breaks *first* because it is so weak, *then* they fall down. Osteoporosis can often be halted by the simple measure of adding calcium to the diet to increase bone density.

According to the U.S. Department of Agriculture, *three out of every ten families have a calcium intake below the recommended minimum.* You probably get enough calcium if you drink a quart of milk a day or eat thirty ounces of cottage cheese or four ounces of hard cheese. Otherwise, researchers believe you should take calcium supplements as a lifelong routine. They are obtainable in any drug and health store.

Bonus benefits from calcium supplements: your cholesterol levels will usually decrease, leg cramps often disappear, there often is a lessening of irritability and fatigue.

Note: Some doctors claim that excessive calcium can cause kidney stones, so those who have a history of kidney stone problems should consult their physician before using calcium supplements. Because of widespread calcium deficiencies and the bad effects on back and bone from such a deficiency, many doctors we talked to recommended that *everyone* over the age of twenty-one take regular calcium supplements. One osteoporosis specialist says she bakes her own bread and adds a cupful of calcium carbonate powder to each eight-pound batch. The taste is undetectable, she says, and offers a good alternate to taking calcium in tablet form.

Pregnant and nursing mothers definitely need calcium supplements, since the developing fetus absorbs so much calcium from the mother's supply during the last three months of pregnancy. Moreover, breast-feeding uses up about 250 milligrams of calcium a day.

Menopausal women often find that calcium can prevent bone loss without the side effects often produced when estrogen is taken to offset bone deterioration after menopause.

Persons who are intolerant of milk and who thus may be deficient in calcium should also pay particular attention to their calcium intake.

Aging people almost always need calcium supplements, doctors say. Not only do they generally take in less calcium in the diet, but as people age, their calcium absorption capacity lessens. "If you read statements that calcium requirements go down with age, this is absolutely untrue," one doctor said. In addition, older people often do not get enough of the exercise that helps prevent the loss of calcium. Diuretics, used for high blood pressure, and other medicines can increase the need for calcium, potassium, and other minerals. One doctor suggested preventing the problem of poor nutrition in old age by starting a nutritional pension plan. Build up a food nutritional program now to pay off later when you need it most.

How You Can Tell If You Have a Calcium Deficiency

In addition to hair testing, your *dentist* may be able to tell you if you have calcium deficiency and impending osteoporosis. It is often the jawbone that first shows signs of demineralization. What's happening there indicates what's starting to happen to the bones all over your body. As bone loses essential calcium, it shrinks bit by bit, until the teeth become loose in their sockets. Sometimes before the teeth become loose, periodontal disease occurs—gums become inflamed, bleed, often begin to recede, exposing the tooth roots. If your dentist finds signs of bone weakening, you may be able to take steps to correct the calcium deficiency before your spinal vertebrae show the same signs of thinning and collapse.

Bones in the fingers show early signs of mineral loss, too. In fact, one team of doctors and dentists from New York devised a method of measuring bone density by taking an X-ray of the middle bone of the little finger.

The encouraging thing is that in both the jawbone studies and the little-finger studies, adding calcium to the diet corrected the bone problems. Patients who showed jawbone deterioration were found to have a deficiency of calcium and an excess of phosphorus in their diet. They were divided into three groups: one took a gram of calcium supplement per day, another added one quart of skim milk to the diet (which supplies about one gram of calcium), and the third group served as a control, making no change in their diet. The two groups taking calcium showed a very significant increase in jawbone density when they were restudied twelve months later.

In the group whose fingers were being studied by X-ray, the doctors selected twelve elderly women aged seventy to eighty-nine, who, as expected, were shown to have a diet deficient in calcium. They were given 750 milligrams of calcium and 375 units of vitamin D (essential for calcium utilization by the bones). Another group of women served as controls and did not receive extra calcium. After three years, measurements showed that the bone density of women receiving the extra calcium had increased so that, even though they were older, *their bones were actually younger.* In those who had not received extra calcium, bone density was even lower than it had been before. The only side effect, the investigators said, was a good one—the women showed a striking decrease in their serum cholesterol levels.

Most investigators said the beneficial effects on the bones usually take at least six months to occur and so urge patients not to become discouraged if they do not see immediate improvement, but to keep up the calcium supplementation on a long-term basis.

Interestingly, another researcher found that bones and their muscles tend to regain strength at the same rate. The protein content of the muscles builds up as the calcium content of the bone builds up. This body wisdom prevents a muscle from being so strong that it could contract and snap the bone it is attached to.

Note: A high protein intake causes calcium to be flushed out of the system, so doctors recommend that people who eat large amounts of protein be especially sure to watch their calcium levels.

Prolonged use of cortisone or its derivatives can also lead to severe calcium loss, to the point that patients frequently develop advanced osteoporosis and run a high risk of bone fracture. Most doctors recommend that anyone taking cortisone should take calcium supplements routinely, along with vitamin D, to prevent the expected bone degeneration.

Bone that is immobilized also loses calcium. Even healthy young persons who have had an arm or leg in a cast for several weeks will have as much as a 50 percent loss of calcium. When the bone is no longer immobilized and is exercised and used for weightbearing, it recovers. (This is why people with osteoporosis are no longer put into braces. Doctors now know that it is not protection, but exercise and calcium that are needed for recovery and to prevent fractures.)

Foods That Are Good Calcium Sources

Green leafy vegetables
Oranges
Pineapples
Milk
Natural cheese
Nuts
Beans

21 What to Expect at the Doctor's Office

WHEN TO GO TO THE DOCTOR

Most people with bad backs do not go to the doctor soon enough. They may have pain in the hip or leg and not even associate it with a back problem. They may think of their problem as a temporary strain instead of a possible sign of a more severe problem. They may get so used to periodic back pain that they accept it as normal.

But the truth is, if a slightly bad back is not attended to, the chances are strong that the condition will get worse. And some back pain can be a sign of serious disease—even cancer—that could be life-threatening if not attended to promptly. Whenever back pain is severe, or even when mild discomfort is constant or frequently reappears, a doctor should be seen for diagnosis and advice.

Always be sure to see a doctor:

1. If backaches don't respond to simple treatment.
2. If backaches become more frequent or are longer-lasting.
3. If backache results from an injury.
4. If there is fever.
5. If there is pain that travels down one or both legs or arms.
6. If there is numbness or tingling in the arms or legs.
7. If the neck is so stiff that the head cannot be lowered toward the chest.
8. If there is any severe limitation of movement.

142

The most ominous signs—i.e., that a backache could be connected to cancer—are a back pain that seems to come on suddenly out of nowhere without injury, continuing pain that is not helped by rest, and pain that is particularly bad in bed at night. If you have any of these symptoms, you should see your doctor today for immediate X-rays and laboratory tests.

SOME MAJOR CAUSES OF BACK PAIN

The major reason that you need to see a doctor if you have severe or persistent back pain is that so many things can be the cause of the pain, some minor and some major, some even life-threatening. Some causes can be sudden and injurious, others can have been acting on the back for years, causing gradual wear and tear until the pain finally becomes disabling.

Here are some of the major causes of back pain that your doctor will have in mind as he examines you and makes his diagnosis:

Sudden twisting of the vertebrae
A blow causing an injury
A fall from a height causing sudden compression of the bones and disks in your spine
Strain from lifting a heavy or awkward object
Sleeping on a poor mattress
Poor standing, sitting, or walking posture
Flabby abdominal muscles
Overweight
Slipped or herniated disk
Birth defect
Infections of the spine or spinal fluid
Kidney trouble
Disorder of the uterus
Prostate trouble
Tumors, both benign and cancerous
Arthritis
Vitamin deficiencies
Metabolic disease
Hormone changes of menopause
Osteoporosis
Strain of muscles during pregnancy

Referred pain from pneumonia
Referred pain from ulcers
Emotional tension
Weakness from poliomyelitis
Cancer that has spread from other sites, especially from the
     lung
Abscess of the spine secondary to a carbuncle, boil, or abscess
Pancreas disease
Circulatory disorders
Muscle spasm
Not enough exercise
Improper exercises
One leg longer than the other
Aneurysm (dangerous ballooning and weakening of an ar-
     tery)
Liver disorders
Gallbladder disease
Disease of the reproductive organs
Improper lifting
Clots in blood vessels
A nerve disorder
Bone disease
Disorders of the feet, such as fallen arches
Improper shoes
Imbalance of muscles of the back and legs

And don't forget that sometimes back trouble doesn't always
show up as pain in the back. It may be felt as pain somewhere else,
such as in the leg or buttocks. This is because the distribution of
nerves as they come from the spinal cord makes the pain feel like
it is coming from the area the nerve serves.

Or conversely, there can be referred pain from another part
of the body which is interpreted as back pain. For example, in
disorders of the gallbladder, which is in the front of the body
under the ribs on the right side of the abdomen, the pain may be
felt in the back under the right shoulder blade.

Dr. Leon Root, orthopedic surgeon at The Hospital for Special Surgery in New York, and author of *Oh, My Aching Back*, tells,
through his own experience, how referred pain works. "I had
suffered for many years with chronic severe back pain but had

conquered it through back-strengthening exercises which I diligently pursued. Then, one day, after a particularly strenuous day in the operating room and in my office, I experienced some rather sharp pain in my right mid-back region. I was sure I had pulled a muscle or strained myself in some way during my day's activities, but I had an even deeper fear that perhaps my old pain was about to reappear.

"My initial reaction was to try to dissipate the pain by moving my arm around. That didn't work. So I exercised my upper back for a few days. This had always been helpful to me in the past when I suffered specific muscle strains, but the pain still did not go away. So then I decided to give my back a few days of rest in the hopes that the pain would subside spontaneously. Still no luck.

"During the following weekend, in fact, my back pain increased in intensity and I began to have a low fever. Finally I did the wisest thing—what I should have done in the first place. I stopped treating myself and visited an internist. He examined me, took X-rays, and discovered that I had a case of viral pneumonia."

DIFFERENT SPECIALISTS AND WHAT THEY DO

Family practitioner. A good bet to start with if you have a back problem since he knows your medical history. Your family practitioner can refer you to a specialist if appropriate.

Orthopedic surgeon. A physician with an M.D. or a D.O. degree, who has spent three to four years in residency in his specialty of treating bone and muscle problems. Although he is a surgeon, he also uses various nonsurgical treatments for the preservation and restoration of the function of the skeletal system, including all bones and joints. Also called orthopedist.

Neurologist. A physician who specializes in the treatment of disorders affecting the nervous system, including the spine and spinal nerves. A neurologist uses both surgical and nonsurgical methods.

Physiatrist. A physician who specializes in physical medicine using physical means for treating disorders. He does not perform surgery. He usually has a non-M.D. physical therapist work with patients to give exercises, heat treatments, ultrasound therapy, etc., and frequently is also involved in rehabilitation medicine to improve and restore function. Also called physiatrician.

Osteopathic physician. A fully trained physician who has gone to a school of osteopathic medicine which awards the Doctor of Osteopathy, D.O., degree rather than the M.D. degree. A D.O. has the same range of rights and responsibilities as an M.D. and may be a general practitioner or a specialist. The difference in osteopathic training is the emphasis on the interdependence of the musculoskeletal, circulatory, and nervous systems and the body organs, and on manipulative therapy as an additional means of diagnosis and treatment. The osteopath (D.O.) also uses drugs, surgery, muscle relaxants, traction, heat and ultrasound and medications for back problems as M.D.s do. D.O.s account for 5 percent of the nation's physicians, and handle 10 percent of all patient visits.

Chiropractor. They have some medical training in special chiropractor schools but do not have a degree in medicine. They use manipulative techniques but cannot prescribe medicines or perform surgery or use other medical techniques that invade the body in any way. Chiropractors believe that misalignments of the vertebrae of the spine can produce a variety of symptoms which may often then be cured or helped by an adjustment to put the bony structures back into their proper alignment. Most, but not all, chiropractors who belong to the International Chiropractors Association (ICA) largely confine themselves to the use of X-rays to locate subluxations and use manual adjustments to correct them. Most of those represented by the American Chiropractic Association (ACA) also use heat, hydrotherapy, ultrasound, and acupuncture, and other devices to aid in diagnosis. At present, chiropractic treatment is reimbursed by Medicaid in twenty-seven states, Medicare in all states, and other government insurance plans in most states. Private insurance companies will also pay bills for back pain treated by chiropractors in most states.

GETTING THE MOST FROM YOUR VISIT TO THE DOCTOR

The more you can tell your doctor, the faster he can make a diagnosis and get started with proper treatment. Don't make him play guessing games if you want an accurate diagnosis and effective treatment aimed at the proper target causing your problem. Getting complete and accurate facts to the doctor is your responsibility as a patient, just as it is your responsibility to ask about any phase of treatment that you do not understand.

When you make your first trip to the doctor to discuss your back problem, have in mind the answers to the following questions, which you will probably be asked.

What is your chief complaint?

What other related or even seemingly unrelated symptoms do you have?

When did you first notice the pain, stiffness, or other symptoms?

Did it start suddenly, or did you gradually become aware of it?

How do you think the problem was produced?

Had you been ill in any other way when it started?

Had you been doing anything unusual before it began that may have led to strain or injury?

When does it bother you most? (in the morning, during the day, at the end of the day, at night, with fatigue, with certain movements, or is it steady and constant?)

Is the pain sharp, aching, dull, throbbing, twinging, burning, cramping, stabbing, shooting?

Is it in one spot or does it seem to spread down the arm or leg or into the buttocks?

Do your symptoms wake you from sleep or keep you from going to sleep? How often?

Have you felt weak or tired, or lost your appetite recently?

Is the pain getting worse, staying the same, or is it less severe than when it started?

Have you changed your style of living or working in the past year?

Have you been under any extra emotional or nervous strain recently?

Does the discomfort seem related to your menstrual period?

Does the pain seem to be related to certain activities, such as going to work, having sexual intercourse, watching television, driving the car, engaging in athletic activities, doing certain work?

Has the pain spread to other joints or areas of your body?

What medications do you take?

Have you ever had a similar problem before? Or any other neck, back, hip, leg, or foot problems?

What treatments did you have for any of these previous problems?

What treatments have you had, if any, for your present problem?

What have you found that helps relieve the problem the most?

Is there anything else you would like your doctor to know about your problem?

In addition to answering these questions, you should also *point* directly to where the pain occurs. Often patients and doctors use different terminology in describing locations.

It sometimes helps to draw an outline of a human figure and then draw a picture of your pain on the figure. Several clinics and pain centers do this so the pain is precisely outlined. Mark an "X" where your pain started. Use an arrow to show the directions in which it spreads. Shade with lines any areas of numbness or pins and needles.

Discuss all your symptoms, even minor ones. This is no time to give in to false modesty, or pretend that you are a superman with no problems.

Tell your doctor everything, even if it seems embarrassing. No matter how embarrassing it may be to you, he or she has heard it before.

Tell as many details and clues as you can so the diagnosis can be made as quickly and accurately as possible.

Don't wait for your doctor to ask you about something; volunteer information. And if you have a hunch as to what the cause of your back problem might be, or a fear about something, discuss it.

Make a list to take with you of all symptoms you want to mention and questions you want to ask, so you don't forget anything. And write down the answers or instructions the doctor tells you, so you don't forget them the minute you walk out of the office.

Work with your doctor, not against him. Your doctor is there to help you. Don't try to challenge him. You gain nothing by fighting him or putting him down.

When your doctor gives you advice, follow it. If he or she gives you medicine, take it. Studies show as many as 60 percent of people go to a physician and then ignore the advice, don't fill prescriptions, don't take medicine properly, or don't finish taking the medicine. (If a treatment does not seem to be working or is causing a side effect, call your doctor so he can alter his instructions. Do not stop taking medicines on your own without letting your doctor know.)

EXAMINATION TECHNIQUES THAT YOUR DOCTOR MAY USE

The doctor will have you undress and examine your back for balance and symmetry. Posture and gait will be checked. You will be asked to bend forward, backward, and sideways and to bend and twist in various directions so that the doctor can check to see if there is any limitation in your motion, or pain with certain movements.

Heat, redness, sweating, patches of hair, swellings, nodules, tenderness will be checked for. Muscles will be checked for weakness or spasm. Reflexes will be checked to determine if there is nerve damage, and your skin will be checked for sensory loss by tiny pinpricks. Urine and blood samples will be taken for laboratory tests.

Osteopathic Palpation

Osteopaths use palpation to a greater extent and in different ways from most other physicians, although many orthopedic surgeons also use their fingers to test for mobility and to feel the condition of underlying tissue. What is osteopathic palpation like?

Dr. William J. Walton, osteopath in Chicago Heights, Illinois, describes some of the techniques in the *Journal of the American Osteopathic Association:*

"In superficial palpation, the operator passes the pads of his fingers lightly up and down over the skin overlying the area being examined, and then increases the depth of his palpating pressure until he can investigate the area further through deep palpation. He checks for swelling, deep muscle tension, bony changes and mobility changes."

He checks flexion by placing the pads of the fingers between the spinous process of the vertebral segments. He checks for separation by comparing the intervals between vertebrae. And he bends the spinal column into different positions to check the vertebrae flexed in different ways.

With these methods, the physician can find temperature changes, muscle tension, tenderness, swelling, reduced elasticity, differences in mobility, bony changes—thereby helping to determine the specific problem areas.

Leg Measurements

The physician usually measures each leg from the iliac spine bump to the malleolus (the big round bone that sticks out on the inside side of your ankle). Discrepancies of more than ¼ inch in leg length can cause pelvic tilt and secondary low back strain. This is one of the most frequently overlooked causes of low back pain, doctors told us, and can easily be corrected in most cases with a simple heel lift.

The doctor will also measure the circumference of each thigh at the midpoint and each calf at the largest diameter. This is to find if there has been any atrophy of the muscles that could indicate a disk problem or other muscle or nerve disorder. Differences of ¼ inch or more in the calves and ½ inch or more in the thighs are considered significant. Smaller differences are disregarded.

The Valsalva Test

This test increases the pressure within the body. To perform the test, you bear down as if you were moving your bowels and at the same time hold your breath. The test is positive if you feel an increase in pain in the neck, upper back, or shoulder. It may indicate a herniated disk or tumor in the spinal canal.

Distraction Test and Compression Test

These two tests are to check for symptoms of osteoarthritis in the neck and to see if neck traction might be of some benefit in relieving the pain.

To perform the *spine distraction test,* the doctor will place the open palm of one hand under the chin and the other hand under the back of the head and gradually and gently lift the head so that the neck is relieved of its weight, widening the spaces between the vertebral joints of the spine and relieving pressure.

In the *compression test,* the doctor presses upon the top of the patient's head to see if there is an increase in pain in the neck, or in the shoulder or arm.

If the tests are positive, it indicates that neck traction might well be beneficial in relieving pain and discomfort.

Electromyography (EMG)

This test may be done to evaluate nerves and muscles by electrically stimulating nerves and then picking up and recording the resulting nerve and muscle electrical activity.

The test takes one to three hours, depending on the number of areas to be tested. It may be done on an outpatient basis or in an overnight stay at a hospital.

Electrodes are placed on the skin. A weak electric current is applied and the resulting electrical activity in the affected nerves and muscles is recorded.

Then needle myography is done by inserting a very thin needle into a muscle a little bit at a time. At each level of insertion measurements are made of the electrical activity of the muscle at rest and as the patient contracts the muscle. Electrical activity is seen on an oscilloscope, and permanent records may be made on paper or tape.

Myelography

This test is usually done only if the physician thinks there is a strong possibility of the need for surgery.

The patient does not eat or drink for several hours before the examination. All jewelry is removed. The examination takes thirty minutes to one and a half hours and is usually done in the radiology department of a hospital.

The patient lies down and a lumbar puncture is performed, inserting a needle between the vertebrae into the spinal canal. A small amount of cerebrospinal fluid is removed, than a contrast medium is injected, and fluoroscope and X-ray pictures are taken of the spinal cord area. The table the patient is lying on is sometimes tilted up or down or at an angle to control where the contrast medium goes in the spinal spaces and to help get better picture angles.

After the test, the head must always be kept higher than the back so the contrast medium does not run into the head. There is sometimes difficulty in passing urine for several hours after the test so the person should drink quantities of fluid to encourage urination.

Any symptoms of pain, nausea, or dizziness or any other reactions during the test or afterward should be reported promptly to the physician.

Several doctors I talked to predicted that myelography will be replaced by a technique called axial tomography, in which scanning of the area is done using X-ray that reveals details of structures by layers of the body, including structures deep within the tissue. Results are laid out by computer for the physician to see and interpret. It is a much more comfortable procedure for the patient than myelography, which usually is extremely uncomfortable.

Bone Scanning

Radioisotope studies of bone tissue are sometimes done. A radioactive chemical is injected into a vein and monitored by a scanner. How and where the bone becomes radioactive makes it possible for the doctor to spot a possible cancer or to determine if an injury to the bone is new or old, often important in lawsuits or workmen's compensation cases.

X-rays

X-ray study will not tell the doctor as much as he might wish it would when it comes to back pain, but it can still be helpful. It can sometimes, but not always, show narrowing of the spaces between the disks of the spine and can reveal osteoarthritic changes. If your doctor takes X-ray pictures, they will be made from several different angles in an attempt to visualize as much as possible of what is going on. X-ray studies are particularly helpful in finding small compression fracture of parts of the vertebrae of the spine. If these are suspected, follow-up X-rays are usually taken six to eight weeks later for comparison, to confirm diagnosis and progress of healing.

Always be sure that a lead apron is placed over your chest and lap when X-rays are taken. Make sure it is done for your children also. Keep still when X-rays are taken so retakes won't be necessary. Children and pregnant women should absolutely avoid X-rays unless there are very urgent reasons for having them taken.

Laboratory Studies

Diagnostic clues can also be found through laboratory tests on the blood. For example, tests for sedimentation rate of the blood and blood cell counts will show if there is an inflammatory process at work in the body; a high uric acid level in the blood indicates gout; other blood tests may indicate the possible presence of arthritis or cancer.

HOW TO FIND OUT WHAT YOUR DOCTOR REALLY MEANS

It is important that you know about your condition in detail and understand exactly what to do. Talk to your doctor. Ask him questions. Take notes on what he says. Make sure you understand his instructions completely. If you don't, ask him to explain.

The following definitions will give the basic parts of the common medical words you might encounter when you talk to your back doctor. By breaking a word down to its component parts you can usually figure out the meaning of most medical words.

When your doctor says . . .	*This is what he really means . . .*
Arthro __	joint
__ itis	inflammation
Arthritis	inflammation of a joint
Costa __	rib
Intercostal	between the ribs
Coxa __	hip
__ algia	pain
Coxalgia	pain in the hips
Myo __	muscle
Myositis	inflammation of muscles
Osteo __	bone
__ otomy	to cut open

Osteotomy	cutting into a bone
Plasty	repair
Arthroplasty	repair of a joint

HOW TO READ THE PRESCRIPTION
YOUR DOCTOR GIVES YOU

Rx   ... *means* ... prescription
Sig   ... *means* ... label
ac   ... *means* ... before meals
ad lib... *means* ... whenever you want
b i d ... *means* ... twice a day
cc   ... *means* ... cubic centimeter
dr   ... *means* ... dram
extr   ... *means* ... extract
gm   ... *means* ... gram
gr   ... *means* ... grains
mg   ... *means* ... milligrams
qd   ... *means* ... every day
q i d ... *means* ... four times a day
q s   ... *means* ... as much as is sufficient
t i d ... *means* ... three times a day

22 Up-to-Date Treatments Your Doctor Might Prescribe

The first recommendations your doctor will give you will probably be simple ones that you can do at home for temporary relief—heat or ice, aspirin, massage, back flattening positions and exercises, all the things we outlined in the earlier chapter on techniques for instant relief. Your physician will also probably prescribe exercises for long-term strengthening of the back, such as the Better Back Ten-Week Exercise Program.

This chapter will explain the entire spectrum of other treatments, old and new, that are currently being used to treat back problems.

When you have a sprain or strain, an injury, or what just seems like a crick in your back, you probably also have muscle spasm, which occurs when the muscles tighten in constant contraction. The symptoms of a spasm include, pain, tenderness, stiffness, and reduced mobility. Usually, if you touch the area gently, the affected muscle seems taut, or extra firm, or there may be swelling. The area is generally very tender, and applying pressure usually makes the pain worse.

Although a muscle spasm is painful, it serves a purpose—to protect the injured area. "The muscles are, in effect, providing an instantaneous internal splint to prevent further aggravations of the trauma," says Dr. Charles V. Heck, executive director of the American Academy of Orthopedic Surgeons.

The first aim of a treatment program for the muscle spasm of sudden backache is to relax these muscles, to get them to return from this contracted state to their length in a normal resting state.

Bedrest is the single most important thing for acute back strain, all doctors agreed. It reduces stress and prevents further strain. "If you suspect an injury or a strain, give it a chance to rest," says Peter Marchisello, an orthopedic surgeon at the Hospital for Special Surgery and Cornell University Medical Center, in New York City. "You give inflammation a chance to subside, contusions a chance to resorb, and any local trauma a chance to recover."

If you have a severe strain, you should remain in bed constantly except for bathroom privileges. To put your back under the least strain and to relax your muscles the most, lie flat on your back or on your side with a pillow under your knees. Try the Flat Back Pelvic Tilt position (Better Back Exercise 3) or any variation of it that makes you most comfortable.

However, doctors caution that rest is a key treatment only for acute conditions, not chronic ones. It's very detrimental to the latter.

MUSCLE RELAXANTS

Muscle spasm often can be relieved by injection of a muscle relaxant or by muscle relaxant pills. These relaxants help break the cycle of muscle spasm that add to back pain. They frequently produce drowsiness, however. Muscle relaxants should not be used more than two or three weeks at the most, experts say. A muscle relaxant does not "cure" backache, but it does help alleviate pain by helping relax the acute local muscle spasm.

Note on tranquilizers: Despite the fact that they are widely used, there is no evidence that tranquilizers are of significant help in managing back pain. Most doctors we talked to felt that tranquilizers were very much over-prescribed and that they were contraindicated for backache unless the person was especially anxious and upset.

TRIGGER POINTS MIGHT BE THE KEY TO CURE

Many times when there is pain, the cause of that pain is somewhere else. A trigger point in the back might cause pain in the hip or arm, for example. Or a trigger point in one part of the back could cause pain in another part of the back. Dr. Janet Travell, of George Washington University School of Medicine in Washington, D.C., and one of President John F. Kennedy's physicians, describes the pain patterns as being so predictable that typical pain patterns and the trigger points that may be causing the pain can be mapped for the entire back.

These highly irritable spots in muscles are among the most important causes of disability from back pain, according to Dr. Travell. Unfortunately, many physicians fail to recognize and treat them, she says, "But if these conditions are promptly diagnosed and effectively treated, patients are spared prolonged disability."

Trigger points can occur in the neck, shoulders, upper and lower back, and hip muscles. They can be caused by constant or acute strain of the muscles or by muscle spasm. They literally can trigger pain by provoking muscle tension or spasm. Trigger points usually appear in your muscles if you let minor episodes of back pain go untreated, and then, once the trigger points have formed, the episodes of pain often increase both in intensity and frequency.

With advancing age, many people accumulate unsuspected latent trigger points, according to Dr. Travell. These may persist for years after seeming recovery from an injury, then may be activated by minor stresses such as periods of immobility, over-stretching of muscles, overuse in repetitive (isotonic) movement or prolonged, fixed (isometric) effort, or even by chilling during fatigue.

Other factors that appear to perpetuate trigger points, she says, are tension, underactive thyroid, estrogen deficiency, chronic infection, anemia, low potassium and calcium levels, and vitamin B-complex and vitamin C deficiencies.

A trigger point can be identified by deep tenderness (local pain) in a hard-feeling band of muscle. If a physician finds a trigger point, he may inject it with a local anesthetic like procaine or with a corticosteroid compound to inactivate the trigger point and stop the pain. Or cooling of the skin (but not the underlying muscle) is done with a vapocoolant spray (Fluori-Methane Spray) while the muscle is gradually stretched. The brief cooling of the skin has a reflex effect on the muscle which allows it to be stretched to its full length. Then the patient can begin an exercise program which maintains the benefits of stretching and increases flexibility of the muscles.

Trigger points and slipped disk are often confused, because like slipped disks, trigger points can cause radiating pain to the back and down the legs or arms. And many times some back-pain sufferer with a trigger point has been incorrectly diagnosed as having intervertebral disk trouble. But trigger points do not cause sensory loss, numbness or weakness, as disks can, unless the taut muscle which harbors trigger points happens to pinch a nerve.

If you have pain and want to determine whether you might have one trigger point or more, study the diagrams of some of the more common trigger points, and have someone push firmly upon the possible location of various trigger points. If it is a trigger point causing pain, the pressure should produce local pain and may even make the muscle jump or twitch. Sometimes, if the point is pushed for several seconds, there will also be referred pain, which reproduces the pain where you usually feel it, proving that this is at least one trouble spot.

The therapeutic use of intermittent cold can produce dramatic relief of pain arising from trigger points, according to Dr. John M. Mennell, former chief of the rehabilitation service, Veterans Administration Hospital in Martinez, California.

A physician often applies cold by playing a thin jet stream of a coolant called Fluori-Methane Spray in even sweeps over the trigger point, then slowly sweeping it toward and over the area of referred pain. Sweeps are repeated in a steady rhythm of a few seconds on and a few seconds off, until all of the skin over trigger-point and referred-pain areas is covered once or twice. While the vapocoolant is being applied, the muscles are gently stretched to promote relaxation and increase the range of motion.

MASSAGE AND PHYSICAL THERAPY

The orthopedic surgeon often has as part of his staff a physical therapist who can give professional deep therapeutic massages to help the back; the therapist can also give ultrasonic therapy (high-frequency soundwaves) or shortwave diathermy treatments (heat created by high-frequency electric currents) or hydrotherapy (with water). Sometimes these therapies are of no benefit, but at times they have been shown to be very helpful in arthritis, bursitis of the shoulder, or in tendinitis, where calcium forms along a tendon.

One study of ultrasound showed that benefits were much greater when low-frequency treatments were used (89,000 waves per second) as opposed to high frequencies of one million waves per second. Apparently the lower frequencies penetrate to a greater depth and so are more effective in relieving pain and stiffness.

Ultrasound can also be used to drive corticosteroid through tissue to the site of injury, a more effective technique than giving corticosteroid by injection. Be sure to get these treatments only from a physical therapist who has been recommended by your doctor.

Fibrositis. This is a special kind of pain that can appear in the back and elsewhere. In this condition, when the skin is gently rolled between the fingers, it may be very sensitive to the touch. Fibrositis is caused by inflammation of the tissues around the muscles. The tenderness will usually disappear gradually if the area is given a gentle pinching massage regularly for several weeks. Sometimes the tender nodules may be injected with a painkilling substance such as procaine.

CORSETS AND BANDS

A physician can make sure you have a well-fitted corset if you need it for temporary relief and stabilization of the back before you begin exercises. Or he may say you only need a wide elastic abdominal binder to provide some support. Most doctors prefer not to use a corset at all unless a patient's abdomen is especially heavy. If corsets are used, physicians caution that support should be only temporary; patients need to build up their own muscle strength for natural body support.

ELECTRICAL STIMULATION

Electrical stimulation is a seldom-used but often effective pain reliever. A battery-powered electric current is applied on either side of a painful area or over the nerve serving the area. The technique is reported to relieve pain in 80 percent of acute pain cases, but in only 25 percent of chronic pain cases. The technique must be administered by specially trained technicians or nurses.

TRACTION

Some doctors consider traction, with the patient stretched in bed, helpful for back pain; others believe the technique is useless except as a device to keep the patient in bed and off his or her back. In a less expensive and less drastic form of traction, which doctors will sometimes recommend, a bar is put across a doorway and the patient hangs by the arms from the bar with feet tucked up. The weight of the body is believed to widen the space between the vertebrae and so remove some pressure from the nerves.

INJECTIONS

As mentioned earlier, the doctor may inject a substance such as procaine into a trigger point, or make an injection directly into the area of a muscle spasm, into the tender pain nodules of fibrositis, or into a joint such as the shoulder joint. Some doctors say they also often can give patients relief by injecting procaine into apparently unrelated scar tissue. Old scars can evidently sometimes set up pain patterns that go to deep tissues and show up as referred pain somewhere else in the body. An injection might be made in an appendectomy scar, for example, and relieve the pain of a frozen shoulder! No one seems to know how it works; the mechanism may be similar to that of acupuncture. In one series of 51 patients a doctor reported that 39 achieved instant relief of pain in one or another part of the body following the injection of a scar.

Doctors sometimes give injections of steroids into a disk to try to cure sciatica, although many physicians warn that this procedure can be dangerous because the needle could cause infection or puncture the wrong area of the spinal cord. Now, as an alternative to this procedure, Dr. John H. Dougherty, Jr., and Dr. Richard A. R. Fraser, of New York Hospital, suggest taking a steroid (they used one called dexamethasone) in high doses that are tapered down over a seven-day period. Relief of pain should occur within the first two days of treatment, the doctors say. In theirs and in other earlier studies, more than 80 percent of patients experienced only mild pain or no pain for an entire year after the medication was given.

Dr. Murray A. Tyber, of Toronto, explained another new

technique of injection at a recent meeting of the American Rheumatism Association. When a bulging nodule of fat on a tendon of a back muscle caused low back pain in his patients, he found it effective to stabilize the nodule by injecting phenol and an anesthetic agent. When a person puts the muscles of certain areas of the back into violent action, such as lifting a heavy object improperly, a tiny wedge of fat, ranging in size from a matchhead to a cherry pit, can come through the muscle connection and cause pain. It is a much more common cause of back pain than is realized, Dr. Tyber says. In 89 patients treated so far, 75 had complete or virtually complete relief of pain. The injections themselves cause pain for one to two days before the back pain is relieved.

ACUPUNCTURE

This technique has been around for thousands of years in China, has been available in France since 1934, and is now available in most areas of Europe, the Soviet Union, and the United States. It consists of inserting very thin needles, so thin they are really wires, into specific points on the skin. Traditional Chinese charts map from 385 to 1,000 points that relate to other specific areas of the body. Incredibly, electronic measurement of the skin's electrical resistance shows differences in these various points, so these areas apparently do exist.

When you have a treatment, the thin wires are inserted into the points that relate to the area of pain that you have. There is no bleeding and, except for a tiny pricking or tingling sensation, no pain on insertion. The needles do not go deep. After several are inserted, you may feel drowsy, and the area usually has a feeling of fullness and numbness which the Chinese call "Da Chi." The needles are usually twirled or given a very slight electrical charge. A treatment takes anywhere from ten minutes to an hour and lasts about twenty minutes on the average.

Before having acupuncture, you should have a thorough examination to determine the cause of your pain. This is to prevent acupuncture from curing a pain that is a warning signal of something serious that should be treated, such as a tumor.

How effective is it in relieving pain? Many doctors claim dramatic relief in many patients even after other treatments have failed to relieve pain over a number of years. Other doctors feel the benefits are overrated. Dr. Jerome H. Modell and a team of investigators at the University of Florida College of Medicine in Gainesville treated 261 patients suffering from various disorders (including arthritis, low back pain, headache, and neuralgia), who had not responded to other methods of pain relief, and found that more than two thirds of them reported their pain was reduced by 50 to 100 percent. However, a month later, only 35 percent said the relief persisted at this level. Only four treatments were given, however, and many acupuncturists feel more treatments should have been given in such difficult cases.

Dr. Louise Wensel, director of the Acupuncture Institute and Research Center, in Washington, D.C., claims an 80 percent success rate in relieving pain of tension headaches, migraines, and low back disorders.

Dr. Ralph Coan, medical director of the Acupuncture Center of Washington, D.C., reports a 65 percent rate of improvement in some 8,000 patients treated over two years.

At Howard University, in Washington, doctors point out that even if acupuncture does not completely alleviate the pain, it frequently reduces pain sufficiently so that the patient with severe problems need no longer be crippled by a need for morphine and other addictive drugs.

The Acupuncture Treatment Group in New York City reports that they are able to produce lasting relief of pain in the back produced by muscle strain or sprain, disk problems, or various types of arthritis after about six to ten treatments. Many patients experience relief of pain during their first treatment, they said, but some need even more than ten. "This varies considerably from person to person," they noted. "A lot depends on the severity of the disease, how long the patient has suffered from it, what drugs have been or are being taken, etc."

At UCLA, Dr. Richard Kroening, of the University's Chronic Pain Clinic, and Dr. David Bresler, director of the Acupuncture Research Project, have given more than 18,000 acupuncture treatments to some 2,000 patients. "It's very clear," they say, "that many low back pain patients should be given acupuncture prior to surgery, and not after all else fails." They found it especially helpful in osteoarthritis.

An adequate trial, most doctors say, is six to ten treatments, two to seven days apart. If you respond, they say, your pain may disappear for days, months or years; there is no way to tell. If you did respond well at one time and the pain later reappears, it usually is helpful to return for a booster treatment.

If a patient with back pain has not had back surgery, acupuncture is more likely to help. Once the patient has had back surgery, pain relief from acupuncture seems to last only a short time.

Most major medical insurance companies will reimburse for acupuncture treatments performed by a licensed acupuncturist, an M.D., or osteopath, and acupuncture services are tax deductible as a medical expense.

If you wish to locate an acupuncture treatment specialist, ask your doctor or local hospital or medical school for a referral. Or check the following two organizations for the name of a qualified acupuncturist in your area: The Acupuncture Information Center, 127 E. 69th St., New York, New York 10021, or The National Acupuncture Research Society, 505 Park Avenue, New York, New York 10022. Be sure to include a stamped, self-addressed envelope.

MANIPULATION

Ever see a dog do a morning stretch and spine extension, or watch a cat lie on its back and flex, extending the spine almost like a snake? That, said one osteopathic physician, is a little bit of what manipulation is all about.

It's designed to rotate and bend the spine at different levels, to move the muscles and bones and joints in ways that relieve pressure and muscle spasm and so relieve pain and stress and congestion and restore proper balance and function. Short muscles are stretched, tight muscles are relaxed. Sometimes you can actually hear a click or feel a sudden snapping into place of a bone or joint as a certain manipulation is performed. It's similar to cracking your knuckles, but on a larger scale.

In one of the most common manipulations for low back pain, the doctor gently rotates your shoulders and hips in opposite directions while you are lying on your back or side with one leg extended and the other bent. Putting traction on the head and neck to separate joints of the cervical spine to relieve neck pain is another frequently used technique.

At one time, only chiropractors and D.O.s used manipulation to treat low back pain and other problems, but now many M.D.s, especially orthopedic surgeons, are taking a look at manipulation and adopting it as another treatment technique in their practice. British orthopedic physician James Henry Cyriax, a teacher at one of the medical association meetings now featuring demonstrations of manipulation to non-osteopathic physicians, says about 50 percent of patients with low back pain can benefit from manipulation. He says he has used or prescribed manipulation for about 40,000 patients in his thirty-five years of practice. He says that about 50 percent of his patients were free of pain after one manipulation. Others needed more than one treatment.

Treatment by manipulation may be effective in early acute episodes of back pain, says Dr. Mark D. Brown, an orthopedic surgeon in Miami. "Mild manipulation often dramatically relieves the acute pain syndrome. Often on manipulation a cartilaginous thud can be heard. . . . The patient may be immediately relieved and grateful." Before manipulation a thorough history and physical exam is necessary.

If manipulation is likely to involve pain or is likely to be particularly difficult, it sometimes is done in the hospital under general anesthesia. Since there are dangers in such a procedure, one should always make sure the person who is to perform the procedure has a good deal of experience in manipulation during anesthesia before proceeding.

Manipulation during general anesthesia, especially of the lumbar spine, should be done only on hospitalized patients who have had the kind of preoperative examinations usually required for major surgery. Neurosurgical or orthopedic consultations are essential, and the patient should have been given fair trial of conservative treatment with little or no progress before manipulation is undertaken.

COCAINE APPLICATIONS

A unique technique being tried by several doctors is putting a little cocaine on the end of a cotton applicator and rubbing it on a nerve center, called the sphenopalatine ganglion, high up in the nose. One doctor who used it said he doesn't know how or why it works, but one man crippled with disk pain got up from the treatment table completely relieved of pain after the procedure. On other patients, however, there was no effect at all.

YOGA

Some doctors recommend yoga exercises for persons with bad backs; others say no, warning that some of the yoga exercises can put undue strain on the back and can do serious harm to a back that is weak. In fact, they say, they get many patients coming to them for the first time with severe back pain because of improper exercising with yoga or other non-medically directed exercise.

Dr. Keith Sehnert, author of *How to Be Your Own Doctor— Sometimes,* finds yoga exercises effective for his own low back pain. Dr. Sehnert, a health consultant in Minneapolis, and much in the forefront of the medical self-care movement, says "A good many physicians, including myself, have taken yoga exercises. My reasons for signing up: patients of mine who'd heard of yoga—or tried it—wanted my medical opinion, and it was embarrassing not to have one.

"I had a personal interest as well. Since falling from a twenty-foot obstacle-course wall while in the Navy in World War II, I've had back problems. I'd been close to surgery twice, but backed away because of possible bad results."

He signed up with a neighbor, who was a yoga teacher. Now, he says, "For the last three years, I've found that if I do my yoga daily, I'm free of back pain."

He still does the Corpse, the Cobra, the Locust, and other yoga exercises on his noon break in the office.

Dr. Sehnert's advice: Don't expect immediate results, because yoga takes months of learning; get competent instruction, and don't try any of the advanced positions before you are ready for them.

We also recommend that if you have back problems of any kind you check with your doctor before considering any yoga exercises, and first try the Better Back exercises in this book, all of which have been approved by back specialists as being safe.

EXTRAORDINARY CAUSES AND TREATMENTS FOR THEM

Perhaps you sit in a draft at work, maybe you have a saggy mattress or a chair that isn't right, or shoes that need replacing.

The wrong bra can be a disaster for a woman with heavy breasts, causing severe upper back pain. Work with your doctor to see if any out-of-the-ordinary things could be causing your backache problem, and learn what to do to correct the situation.

Short-seated

In an earlier section we described what to do for the short leg syndrome—backache caused because one leg is a bit shorter than the other, perhaps only ¼ to ½ inch. But some persons spend more time sitting than standing, and their problems may be an uneven pelvis. Dr. David Heilig, of the Philadelphia College of Osteopathic Medicine, says the answer to this is to put lifts under one buttock to level out how you sit. A pad should be used on the smaller side of the pelvis, he says, and can be as simple as a small magazine put under the buttocks when the patient sits. You can also sew a felt or leather pad into the lining of pants. Some patients permanently attach a pad to one side of their car seat or chair at work.

Any lift should be carefully supervised because of the body's ability to adapt or compensate. Done incorrectly it might create a problem in some other part of the spine and body, Dr. Heilig says.

Fat Wallets Can Cause a Pain

If you have pain in the hip, upper leg, or buttocks, your wallet may be too thick.

Case histories of men who have pain from carrying overly fat wallets in hip pockets are described in the *Journal of the American Medical Association* by Dr. Elmar G. Lutz, of Passaic, New Jersey.

One man who traveled constantly by auto had been troubled for fourteen months by "sciatica," before his doctor noticed the wallet he carried on the painful side. It was 1½ inches thick, packed with credit cards.

"Wallectomy"—transferring the wallet to an inner coat pocket—gave complete relief, the doctor said.

HOW TO RESUME ACTIVITY FOLLOWING A BACK PROBLEM

Don't rush your return to full activity. Give your back as much rest as it seems to need. Your recovery will be faster in the long run. Resume activities gradually and cautiously. Any strenuous activity now can bring the problem back and delay recovery.

Start gentle stretching exercises and back-building exercises as outlined in the Better Back Program.

Practice good posture rules and advice on driving and lifting as outlined in other sections of this book.

Avoid fatigue.

Avoid lifting of any kind. Baby yourself for as many weeks as necessary, and let someone else do all the lifting and heavy work.

23 What Every Back Sufferer Needs to Know about Medicines

WARNING: PAINKILLERS

Many painkiller medicines can be addictive. Don't take medicines without consulting a physician. Don't take medicines if you don't really need them. Don't take them for a longer time than you have been instructed. Get off them as soon as you can.

If you have back pain when you are pregnant, under no circumstances should you take any medicine without consulting a physician, and even then you should take something only if there is a serious need. Most medicines, even something as simple as aspirin, are transmitted to the developing fetus, and many of them, even in small doses, can cause lifelong damage.

Remember that any painkilling drug can be dangerous when taken carelessly. Do not take more medicine than your doctor prescribes, and keep all pill bottles out of the reach of children. Painkillers or other back medicines may be powerful enough to kill a child if taken in quantity.

Which Painkillers Are Best?

According to a study by Dr. C. G. Moertel of the Mayo Clinic, the old standby, aspirin, is still the best among ordinary medicines. Dr. Moertel reported in the *New England Journal of Medicine* in 1972 that a typical dose of regular aspirin (two 5-grain tablets) was better than other pain-relievers evaluated, including codeine, Darvon, Talwin, acetaminophen, and phenacetin. Aspirin is especially good for rheumatoid pain because it acts against inflammation as well as against pain.

Other factors to be considered. Some people are allergic to aspirin and therefore should use non-aspirin painkillers such as Tylenol.

Which Painkillers Are Least Irritating?

A report given at the annual meeting of the Arthritis Foundation showed that, of arthritis drugs tested for their effect on the stomach, ibuprofen (at a dose of 1,660 mg.) was least damaging to the stomach, followed by naproxen (at a dose of 500 mg.), indomethacin, naproxen (750 mg.); the most damage was done by aspirin.

IF YOU TAKE ASPIRIN . . .

Aspirin relieves pain, reduces fever and inflammation, and is cheap, but it can cause side effects, acting as an anticlotting agent, thus often causing stomach bleeding or aggravation of ulcers.

Doctors recommend these rules concerning aspirin: Always take with a full glass of water, and even better, to prevent stomach irritation, chew or crush them before swallowing with water or juice. Do *not* take aspirin (or products like Alka-Seltzer that contain aspirin) if you have stomach distress. Do *not* take it during pregnancy, especially the last three months. Do *not* take it if it gives you stomach upset or if you have an ulcer. Do *not* mix it with beer, wine, or liquor (the mixing increases stomach irritation). Do *not* take it if you are taking other medicine for arthritis, for thinning the blood, or for diabetes. Keep aspirin out of the reach of children; an overdose can kill.

Those doctors tuned in to nutrition also recommend that anyone taking heavy doses of aspirin take vitamin C supplements. Aspirin depletes this vitamin from the body and lowers resistance to a number of diseases, they said.

We also learned that aspirin can sometimes contribute to deafness. The occurrences are rare, usually when people are taking large amounts over long periods, and only in certain people who are sensitive. But if at any time when you are taking aspirin you have ringing of the ears or loss of hearing, call your doctor immediately. If you immediately stop taking aspirin, your hearing will return to normal.

Aspirin can also cause hypoglycemia (a fall in blood sugar), according to Dr. Christopher D. Saudek, director of clinical research at Cornell University Medical College in New York. Many times when an older patient has a sudden change in mental status and the occurrence of a little stroke is suspected, the real cause is a sudden drop in blood sugar caused by large amounts of aspirin, Saudek says. In the journal *Emergency Medicine,* he urged doctors to watch for the condition saying it "is probably a lot more common than is generally realized."

IF YOUR DOCTOR GIVES YOU A PRESCRIPTION FOR CORTISONE . . .

Be sure to tell him if you have a history of tuberculosis or ulcers; cortisone or cortisone products should then not be given.

If you have a persistent backache when you are taking any corticosteroid products, the chances are you are getting osteoporosis, often a side reaction to taking these drugs. Be sure to tell your doctor immediately so he can begin to give you calcium supplements to counteract the problem. Many doctors we talked to said they believe that calcium should always be given with cortisone to *prevent* the bone changes and backache from occurring.

IF YOU TAKE D-PENICILLAMINE . . .

You must keep in close contact with your doctor, always checking back with him or her at the times your doctor suggests for follow-up, because this medicine causes many side effects and must be watched closely. "Go low, go slow" says Dr. David Cooley, rheumatology specialist at the University of Nebraska College of Medicine in Omaha, meaning the dosage should be started at a very low level and be only slowly and gradually built up. In fact, he says penicillamine (*different* from penicillin) should not be used unless all conventional therapies have failed. Typical side effects include nausea, skin rash, mouth sores, and kidney damage.

DMSO

DMSO, short for dimethyl sulfoxide, has been shown to reduce pain and increase joint mobility in many persons with osteoarthritis. It has the unique property of being absorbed almost instantly through the skin to the bloodstream, thus going quickly throughout the body. Research reports indicate DMSO is also effective for reducing pain and swelling in bursitis, tendinitis, sprains, and strains; stimulating healing of open wounds and burns, even when infection is present; clearing up skin ulcers and stiff tissues of scleroderma; relieving pain of shingles and bedsores.

In the United States, DMSO is used primarily in a limited number of medical centers for special problems or on an experimental basis. But it is becoming widely used as an underground medicine, since you can buy it freely in Canada, Japan, Mexico, and many European countries, where it is used frequently by physicians. And since the medicine is approved for use in dogs and horses, some veterinarians have been known to order for doctors and friends.

To use DMSO, you simply dab it on the skin with cotton, and then stay away from friends—it works well but smells terrible.

We interviewed several doctors who used DMSO on back patients when the substance was available, and they all reported good results with it. One New Jersey physician says he had "terrific results" with DMSO for bursitis pain of the shoulder. He also reported good experience using DMSO as a base to carry topical steroids quickly into deep tissue to help various back problems.

NEW NATURAL PAINKILLER

A substance found naturally in the human body, in the pituitary gland, may be available in the future for relieving pain and for treating narcotic withdrawal symptoms. The substance, called endorphin, is similar to morphine but is not addictive, researchers say.

The substance is now being synthesized chemically for cheaper production and use in early clinical trials. Cooperative studies at the University of California (San Francisco) and at Salk Institute in La Jolla show that endorphin secreted by the body produces pain relief during electrostimulation of the brain.

The substance produced in the brain apparently acts as a natural built-in painkiller. Researchers believe the amount released in the bloodstream may explain why different people have different threshold levels for pain. And it might also explain the "placebo effect"—that no matter what treatment is given for pain, including sugar pills, 33 percent of people will feel better. Researchers now hope to come up with better ways to increase production of one form of endorphin, called enkephalin, to reduce pain naturally. One medicine, called D-phenylalinine (DPA) already looks promising. It produces neither addiction nor sedation and apparently needs to be taken only once a month. Used so far on only eleven patients at Chicago Medical School, it produced a marked decrease in pain or total relief of pain in nine. Plans for a large clinical trial are now underway.

NEW DRUG FOR MUSCLE SPASM

A new muscle relaxant called Flexeril has been announced by Merck, Sharp, and Dohme Research Laboratories. It has just been introduced in the United States, Canada, Puerto Rico, and several other countries.

Major use. For the treatment of acute painful muscle spasm caused by back strains and sprains, whiplash and other back, neck, and muscle problems. The drug abolishes excessive muscle contraction—spasm—but leaves motor control untouched, so that a person can take the drug for spasm but still be able to walk about or go back to work.

It is usually used for one to two weeks, and in conjunction with rest and physical therapy.

Side effects. Some drowsiness, dry mouth, occasional dizziness.

GEROVITAL

For the past twenty years, thousands of patients have flocked to clinics in Europe to receive treatments with the controversial Romanian "youth drug" called Gerovital. It is a mixture of procaine (Novocain) and several other substances that the developers of the drug claim is effective in treating depression and memory loss, as well as arthritis and osteoporosis.

Actually there are two forms of the drug: KH-3, developed by Dr. Fritz Widemann, of West Germany, which is one of the top ten over-the-counter sellers in West Germany; and Gerovital H-3, developed by Dr. Ana Aslan, of Romania, which is sold in Switzerland and in Romania, and is given to patients through gerontology clinics set up on farms and in factories across the country. Both are sold in Great Britain. The best results reportedly come from the Romanian version, which is usually given in three injections a week for four weeks, repeated in two weeks for patients past sixty, in two months for those thirty-five to sixty. Simple procaine without the various additions in H-3 seems to have no effect.

At first put down by United States doctors, the two drugs are now being tested by at least five research groups here. So far the tests look promising.

TEN WAYS TO PROTECT YOURSELF FROM SIDE EFFECTS OF DRUGS

There is always the chance that adverse reactions will occur with any drug. Here are ways to protect yourself.

• Always tell a new physician of past drug reactions, even if they were mild. The next one may be more severe. Tell him or her of any medicine you are taking, even something as simple as aspirin or sleeping pills.

• Any time a label is missing, a medicine turns color, is congealed, has started to crumble, or smells like vinegar, throw it out. Always discard medicines on their expiration date.

• When your doctor prescribes a drug, ask the name of the drug and what it is supposed to do. Make sure you understand how and when the drug should be taken, what side effects you should be especially alert for and report. Ask what precautions should be observed while taking the medicine, if it will make you too drowsy to drive a car or operate machinery, if certain foods or activities or other medications should be avoided.

• Ask when you should report back to the doctor. Know if the prescription should be refilled.

Note: You may have more tolerance for pain in the morning than in the evening. So found Dr. Eugene Rogers, chairman of rehabilitation medicine at Chicago Medical School, and psychologist Dr. Barry Vilkin. They believe the differences in pain thresholds are due to biological cycles that everyone experiences on a daily basis. Perhaps you can cut down on pain medicines in the morning.

SOME POSSIBLE SIDE EFFECTS TO BE ALERT FOR

Call your doctor if you are taking medicine and any of the following signs of a reaction occur.
Dizziness
Nausea and vomiting
Wheezing or shortness of breath
Inflammation of the eyelids or reddening of the eyes
Skin rash, itching, or hives
Blood in the urine or stools
Diarrhea
An agitated or upset emotional state
Headache
Ringing in the ears

DO YOU HAVE ANY OF THESE CONDITIONS?

Before you take any medicine, you should tell your doctor if you have any of these conditions that could lead to side effects or necessitate changes in dosages: drug addiction; epilepsy; glaucoma or other eye disorders; heart trouble; peptic ulcer; diabetes; asthma, emphysema or breathing disorder; kidney trouble including kidney stones; liver disease.

ASK THAT YOUR MEDICINES BE LABELED AS TO CONTENTS

Know exactly what your medications are; do not accept an unknown remedy without explanation. To be an intelligent patient you need to know what you are taking, and why.

The information can also be invaluable if you change physicians, if a warning is issued against the use of a particular drug (so you would know if you are taking it), and if a child accidently swallowed pills and you need to be able to identify the pills to know what should be done.

BEWARE OF MIXING MEDICINES

At any time you are given a prescription, your doctor should ask if you are taking any other medication in case there is a conflict. If he doesn't do so, volunteer the information yourself. Many things can go wrong when medicines are mixed.

If you are taking calcium, and your doctor then prescribes tetracycline for an infection, be sure to remind him of the calcium. It can interfere with the action of the antibiotic.

If you are diabetic, remember that insulin can be neutralized by aspirin and some arthritis medicines. Aspirin can also counteract gout pills and some of the new arthritis drugs, and it can abet blood-thinning by anticoagulants.

If you mix arthritis medications like Azolid, Butazolidin, indocin or Sterazolidin with anticoagulants like Coumadin, Dicumarol, Panwarfin or Sintrom, blood-thinning can be increased so much that there is great danger of internal hemorrhaging. Some strong arthritis medicines also decrease the effectiveness of birth control pills, so be sure you are safe.

So if you are taking any medicine, for your back or anything else, don't add a second medicine without checking with your doctor.

WATCH WHAT YOU EAT AND DRINK

Some foods can be deadly when combined with medicines. If you are taking tranquilizers, do not eat chicken livers, bananas, avocado, canned figs, broad beans, soy sauce, yogurt, Camembert, Gruyère, Cheddar or American cheese or sour cream or drink Chianti. They could kill you.

Some herb teas can change the rate of absorption of certain medicines, making them ineffective, as can nicotine from cigarettes.

Don't drink alcohol when you are taking drugs either. The mixture, if it involves a barbiturate, for example, can kill you. And if you take large doses of aspirin, be aware that both alcohol and aspirin depress the central nervous system, so their effect is additive and dangerous, and together they also make your stomach supersensitive to damage.

THREE POTENTIALLY ADDICTIVE AND LETHAL DRUGS TO GUARD AGAINST

In a special study requested by President Carter, three groups of drugs have been named dangerous by the National Institute of Drug Abuse and the Food and Drug Administration. They are sleeping pills, tranquilizers, and amphetamines. The government agencies say doctors prescribe the drugs too easily, often for longer periods than they should, or for problems that may not even be helped by such drugs. And the government claims that patients who use the drugs for a long time risk developing emotional dependence or physical addiction, possibly leading to death.

Sleeping pills and tranquilizers are the most prescribed drugs in the world, government officials say, with sleeping pills alone accounting for 27 million prescriptions last year—or about 1 *billion* doses. One kind, barbiturates, were implicated in almost 5,000 deaths. The problem is that there is a rather narrow margin of safety between the minimal dose needed for treatment and a dose that can kill. Not realizing this, people may feel that if one pill works well, more will work better, or they may wake up in the middle of the night and take extra pills while half asleep. Alcohol or other drugs can combine with them to increase their effect, causing coma or death.

Amphetamines, often prescribed to help people lose weight by curbing the appetite, can easily be habit-forming and, just like the sleeping pills and tranquilizers, lead the user to try higher doses, as tolerance to the drug develops. Occasionally, they have been used in connection with weight loss for back problems. Diet experts like Dr. Robert Atkins, with whom I co-authored *Superenergy Diet,* also warns that amphetamines hinder weight loss in the long run, having a rebound action that makes it harder to lose weight than previously.

So protect yourself—don't use these drugs unless you and your doctor consider it absolutely necessary, and never take them for long periods or in larger doses than your doctor prescribes.

Common Brand Names to Watch for

Barbiturates. Amytal, Butisol, Carbrital, Luminal, Nembutal, Seconal, Tuinal.

Benzodiazepines. Dalmane, Librium, Libritabs, Serax, Tranxene, Valium.

Amphetamines. Benzedrine, Desoxyn, Dexedrine.

Others. Doriden, Equanil, Meprospan, Miltown, Noctec, Noludar, Quaalude, Placidyl, Parest, Somnos and Sopor.

HOW TO SAVE MONEY WHEN YOU BUY MEDICINES FOR YOUR BACK

Check mail-order discount drugs. Many companies now sell drugs at discount by mail.

Check special organizations. The Retired Teachers Association, the American Association of Retired Persons, and some insurance companies offer drugs at reduced prices.

Check your insurance policy. About 35 percent of people have medical insurance that covers medicines—but many don't use it.

Ask your doctor for free samples. They are often left by detailmen from pharmaceutical companies.

Buy in large quantities where possible. Ask the druggist whether a particular item is cheaper in quantity. However, be sure to check on how long a medicine will last and determine whether you will use the larger quantity before it begins to deteriorate.

Store drugs properly. If directions say to keep a medicine in the refrigerator, keep it there. Keep caps on tightly to prevent evaporation.

Do comparison shopping. Ask at various drugstores for prices on medicines that you use frequently.

Discuss the price of medicine with your doctor. Many doctors have already compared the costs of medicines in the local drugstores.

Use generic names when you can. Sometimes a specific brand name is the best, and your doctor may definitely want it for you, but when brands are alike, ordering the prescription by the generic name can save you money. Check with your doctor.

Ask your doctor to use the new **Physician's Guide to Prescription Prices.** It lists every prescription drug and its average cost. When two drugs are equally satisfactory, he can see which is most economical.

Ask your pharmacist. He can usually recommend the least expensive brand to do the job.

24 Back Schools You Can Attend

Something new has started in many parts of the world—back schools. They are centers where people can go to learn new posture and living habits and do exercises to strengthen their backs. Their very existence and their popularity is evidence of the spread of back problems everywhere, in a virtual epidemic.

One of the most extensive programs is in Toronto, Canada, where back schools are held at medical centers throughout the city in one coordinated program designed to improve back problems and cut the medical costs of the citizens of Toronto. Patients are instructed in proper posture, lifting techniques, work habits, and exercises for back-strengthening as well as on the emotional aspects of chronic pain. The program has become so popular that units have now been opened throughout Ontario, and educational programs have been set up for industries.

At the University of Iowa, the department of orthopedics is setting up a control center for research and training in the treatment of the back, and it plans satellite treatment centers and back schools in the communities where patients would go for help after evaluation in the main center. Feminist centers are setting up schools and workshops in many cities.

Back schools are being set up in Europe also, the most well-known one being at the Institute of Rehabilitation Medicine at Sahlgren Hospital, in Göteborg, Sweden. There patients go for four workshop lessons plus instruction in exercises in the center's swimming pool. In addition to the classes (and examinations to make sure patients have really learned basic principles), a physiotherapist visits each patient's work-site for an hour to analyze working conditions.

In other instances, such as at the Crozer-Chester Medical Center, in Chester, Pennsylvania, a back school is held in conjunction with a back pain clinic that covers medical diagnosis and treatment. There, director Dr. Bernard E. Finneson says patients can get individual medical care, as well as receiving the benefit of class instruction as part of a group.

At the University of Miami School of Medicine a back school is being set up as part of the back clinic, and there is also a Spine Research Center, where research is being done on the *causes* of spinal disorders and the actual origins of the pain involved, as well as on diagnosis and treatment.

THE Y PROGRAM

Probably the most widespread program is that offered in YMCAs and YWCAs in many cities throughout the country. Called "The Y's Way to a Healthy Back," it is a six- or twelve-week program, which already has more than 20,000 graduates and claims an 88 percent improvement record among its participants.

Classes are held for an hour twice a week plus daily homework and are limited to fifteen men and women. Doctor's consent is needed. Classes are taught by physical therapists who were trained by local back specialists.

Tests are given to discover muscular weakness or malfunction. Then students are taught a series of progressive exercises to relax and loosen muscles and strengthen and provide flexibility, as well as doing prescribed homework assignments.

Fee: $30 for non-Y members, $20 for members. Check your local Y.

BOARDER BACK SCHOOLS

For the person with a more serious problem some medical centers and institutions have live-in schools. At the Villa Rosa Medical Center, for example, the University of Texas Health Science Center at San Antonio has set up a program where patients come to live for four weeks. The program is specifically designed to enable the person with debilitating low back pain to learn to cope with himself, his job, and everyday living.

The program includes everything medically acceptable in a package approach to treat the patient, explains Dr. Kenneth Washburn, associate professor of physical medicine and rehabilitation and director of the program.

Candidates for the program must be referred to the clinic by a physician, must be ambulatory, and must remain as in-patients for four weeks.

Those accepted for admission cannot be using any injectible medication and must be willing to participate wholeheartedly in the program, according to Washburn. Once admitted, the patient undergoes an extensive evaluation of physical status, activity levels, and medications. A team approach for instruction and rehabilitation combines a program of rehabilitative medicine, behavior modification, biofeedback, counseling, medication, and exercise. Exercises are designed for each individual, and the patient proceeds at her or his own rate until she or he reaches a level equivalent to that of an able-bodied person. Exercises in a swimming pool allow patients to build up muscles using the buoyancy of the water.

"Essentially, our program proposes to help the patient cope with his pain, understand the structure of the spine and causes of back problems, teach self-treatment methods, and allow him to become functional again," Washburn says.

There are back schools at Parkland Memorial Hospital and Caruth Memorial Rehabilitation Center, both in Dallas, Texas. Both in-patients and out-patients participate in the schools, depending on the severity of their problems; the in-patients have an all-day program. Seven o'clock in the morning finds them walking or jogging. After breakfast they swim in a heated pool, do exercises, attend pain-management classes, have group work with a psychologist, work with the physical therapist, and relax with biofeedback. In between they are expected to spend at least four and as much as six hours in relaxation exercises using individual tapes.

A typical stay is two to three weeks at $1,000 a week. "In most cases, the cost is borne by insurance companies, which are gambling a few thousand dollars versus years and years of repeated operations and chronic office visits," a school spokesman said. Both vocational and retraining opportunities are also available.

Most important, according to medical director Dr. David Selby, are the behavior changes that the health team works toward during a patient's stay.

"We want patients to become receptive to new ways of looking at things, to learn new ways of doing things, to affect changes in their life-styles that will be positive as far as pain is concerned," he says.

In the back school, patients learn to relax, to massage the muscles that are causing much of their pain, even to growl to relieve the tension. And while the medical doctors are working with the patients to cut their drug dependence, the psychologist is working with them to master substitute techniques for managing their pain that they can use for the rest of their lives. Sometimes patients' spouses are invited to the school to learn proper massage techniques.

25 When Arthritis Gets to Your Back

There are many different kinds of arthritis. They may have different symptoms and may vary greatly in severity from one person to another. Arthritis can occur in children as well as adults.

And many things mimic arthritis. So if you suspect you have arthritis, it is essential for you to see a doctor to get a proper diagnosis and find a treatment that is right for you.

The following are the three most common types of arthritis that can affect the back.

RHEUMATOID ARTHRITIS

This form of arthritis can occur at any time, from childhood to old age. Women are affected two to three times more often than men.

It usually begins with swelling and congestion of the joints of the fingers and toes. You may have muscle pain and stiffness, numbness and tingling of the hands and feet, fatigue, weight-loss, and feel sick and stiff all over even before joint symptoms appear. As the disease progresses, it spreads to other joints—the wrists, elbows, knees, shoulders, hips, and spine. There is often muscle stiffness, particularly in the morning or after periods of inactivity. Joint pain, swelling, and muscle stiffness usually become worse with time.

In rheumatoid arthritis, symptoms seem to come and go.

There are remissions, then recurrences of the symptoms, so the patient and the doctor simply cannot predict the pattern of the disease at any time. During active attacks, there is often fever.

Juvenile Rheumatoid Arthritis

Also known as Still's disease, this form of rheumatoid arthritis especially affects children under age five, and generally involves the spinal column of the neck. The cause is unknown. It is often difficult to detect. See a doctor if your child shows a reluctance to crawl or walk, or cries when limbs are moved. Other symptoms include a high fever, rash, and involvement of the wrist or finger joints as well as the neck. There may be only one occurrence of the problem, or it may continue persistently.

Children with juvenile rheumatoid arthritis are treated similarly to adults, except that corticosteroids should not be used because of their tendency to retard growth. Indomethacin and phenylbutazone also are not recommended for children. The disease often becomes inactive when the child reaches puberty.

ANKYLOSING SPONDYLITIS (Marie-Strümpell's disease)

This also is a progressive inflammatory form of arthritis, and attacks the back in particular. It used to be called rheumatoid spondylitis. It generally affects persons between the ages of twenty and forty, and was once considered ten times more common in men than women, although it is now considered to have the same frequency in both.

The onset may be slow or sudden. Any history of repeated backaches or pain in the buttocks and thighs should always make one consider the possiblity of ankylosing spondylitis, and X-rays should be taken.

There is some genetic disposition to the disease. African blacks seldom get it; North American Indians frequently do.

Early-morning pain and stiffness are characteristic. Stiffness in the lower back often lasts several hours in the morning, then is relieved, but returns in the evening. There is sometimes pain and stiffness in the middle of the night. As the disease progresses, there is increasing stiffness of the back, unless physiotherapy is instituted. Strangely, spondylitis is often associated with pain and discomfort of the eyes and with ulcerative colitis. X-ray will usually reveal a specific diagnosis within six months of the onset of pain.

Sign: Often if a person has had ankylosing spondylitis for a long time, he cannot bend forward farther than to touch the knees. Also with arms outstretched, the distance from fingertips to fingertips is greater than the person's height. (Normally the measurements are equal.)

Sometimes the disease mysteriously becomes inactive ten to fifteen years after onset, leaving a rigid, stiff spine but little or no pain. Sometimes breathing is restricted and emphysema can result, so breathing exercises should be learned.

OSTEOARTHRITIS

This arthritis is completely different. It is not inflammatory, so the person does not have bouts of fever and inflammation as in the first two kinds of arthritis discussed. Osteoarthritis is the most common form of arthritis, and is a frequent component of aging, usually causing symptoms only after the age of fifty. But it can appear earlier in a joint that has been damaged by disease or injury. The cartilage of the joint—usually a large joint—breaks down, and bony growths form at the edges of the joint, making it swollen and knobby, a kind of exaggeration of the natural aging process of the joints. In the finger joints these growths are called Heberden's nodes. If only one joint is affected, it is usually because of an injury that occurred to a joint or a neighboring joint some years before. Otherwise the breakdown is most likely to occur in weight-bearing joints or joints subjected to a lot of use and strain—the hips, neck, knees, fingers, and back. Most people over age fifty have some osteoarthritis, but only about 5 percent have serious, disabling symptoms. Symptoms are particularly common in people who have engaged in years of heavy labor, and in people who are very overweight.

Pain usually occurs after the joint has been used; it is relieved by rest. As the disease progresses, pain increases and movement may become limited.

Early signs of osteoarthritis: Before there is pain, a person developing osteoarthritis may walk with one foot turned outward as the body attempts to compensate for early stiffness of the hip. When pain first appears, the person may begin to walk stiffly and awkwardly.

BEST TREATMENTS TO TRY FOR ALL KINDS OF ARTHRITIS

Stay slim to reduce the burden on joints.

Get plenty of rest, especially when there is inflammation or fever. Complete bed rest is recommended in a severe attack of rheumatoid arthritis with fever, but usually is not needed for osteoarthritis. The more severe the condition, the more rest is needed, but time in bed should be kept to a minimum, especially in older people who are in danger of developing weakness, bed-sores, or blood clots from inactivity. (If long bed rest is needed during an acute attack, foot and leg exercises should be done every day.)

If a joint is inflamed, as in an acute attack of rheumatoid arthritis, the joint should be rested and the patient should not put any weight on the joint.

Despite the need to rest painful joints, plenty of exercise is essential to prevent muscle atrophy and joint stiffness. Be sure to exercise when there is no inflammation (sex is okay too, in fact, it is beneficial, studies show). Exercise increases flexibility of joints, builds up supporting muscle, and corrects posture weaknesses. Many patients claim relief from pain for the first time after taking up active sports and vigorous exercise. Check with your doctor. Even if a joint is painful, it should be put through its entire range of motion twice daily to prevent later stiffness or contracture and to maintain flexibility. Exercises in a warm-water pool are often helpful.

General rule for exercise: It should restore mobility and strength with the least possible pain.

Other Aids to Arthritis Back Pain

Have gentle manipulation done periodically.

Establish good posture and breathing habits.

Use a firm mattress.

Use heat treatment two to three times a day: hot tub baths, hot moist towels, heat lamps, heating pad, paraffin baths.

Or try cold compresses or ice. Latest results from Temple University Medical School show that in some people ice packs produce longer relief from pain and better function than does heat.

Have a regular massage and physiotherapy.

Do exercises from the Better Back Program and those recommended by your doctor.

Increase your intake of vitamins and minerals, with extra calcium.

Try a hot, dry climate.

Lie flat on your back for thirty minutes in the middle of the day.

Try rubber heels on shoes; they sometimes help reduce jarring to the spine.

Avoid strenuous work that involves heavy lifting, carrying, and straining. But also try to avoid occupations that require long hours of uninterrupted sitting; and if you can't, be sure to get up and have mild exercise frequently.

A surgical corset will sometimes give temporary relief of back pain.

Try wearing a body suit at night.

Acupuncture has sometimes been reported to be beneficial.

Different Aids for Different Stages

Some treatments work for some forms of arthritis and not for others, or for some people and not for others; and some things work at one stage of the disease and not at other stages.

The first thing for you to do is always see your doctor for proper diagnosis and advice on the best treatment for your case. With his advice for your particular problem in mind, you can then experiment yourself with the various possibilities that have helped others.

FINDING YOUR WAY THROUGH THE MAZE OF DRUGS FOR ARTHRITIS

Aspirin (especially when compounded with magnesium or copper), injections of gold salts, phenylbutazone, antimalarial drugs, indomethacin, and corticosteroids are the most standard drug treatments. (Do not mix these drugs because of possible interaction.)

Aspirin. This is the most common treatment, often used in doses as high as three to four tablets every four hours. It often reduces joint swelling as well as alleviating pain. If aspirin affects hearing or causes dizziness, the dose should be reduced. To decrease gastrointestinal effects, take aspirin after meals—not before, or after taking an antacid.

Corticosteroids. Injected into the joints, they give relief in about half of patients, but frequent injections should be avoided. With cortisone pills, take vitamin D and calcium to keep bones strong, and make sure medication is reduced slowly, not all at once.

Phenylbutazone (Butazolidin). This drug is sometimes used to treat ankylosing spondylitis; however, there often are side effects, so it should be used at the lowest possible dosage. It is also effective in osteoarthritis, gout, and bursitis. Side effects include irritation and ulceration of the upper gastrointestinal tract, water retention, skin rash, and upsets in the bone marrow. Patients taking it should have frequent blood counts. Phenylbutazone should be taken with meals or milk and should be accompanied by antacid therapy. It should not be taken with coumarin or other blood-thinning drugs. It should be used only with caution in heart patients.

Indomethacin (Indocin). This is somewhat less potent, and also less toxic, than phenylbutazone. Most doctors prefer a trial with aspirin or indomethacin before resorting to phenylbutazone. Indomethacin is beneficial in about 50 percent of patients with rheumatoid arthritis. It is not approved for use in osteoarthritis (but is sometimes used), except for osteoarthritis of the hip, for which it often provides dramatic relief. It is also effective in the treatment of ankylosing spondylitis and gout. During the early phases of indomethacin treatment, some patients experience nausea or headache; however, with continued use, these symptoms tend to clear, or the dosage can be started low and then increased. Indomethacin, like aspirin and phenylbutazone, irritates the upper gastrointestinal tract, and the same precautions should be used. Long-term use of indomethacin may be associated with eye problems, so patients receiving it should have an examination by an ophthalmologist every six to twelve months. It should not be used in children, pregnant women, nursing mothers, patients with ulcers, or patients allergic to aspirin.

Mental alertness and motor coordination may be reduced, so persons taking the drug should not drive or perform other potentially dangerous activities requiring concentration.

Always take indomethacin with food or immediately after meals to decrease stomach upset. Begin by taking one-half pill, then gradually working up to the recommended dosage. Stop taking the medicine if you develop headaches or blurred vision. If you take indomethacin for a prolonged period, have an occasional blood test to make sure you are not developing anemia as a side effect. As soon as the flare-up of your arthritis or other back pain has subsided, call your doctor so that you can taper off the drug as soon as possible.

HOW TO HELP PREVENT DEFORMITIES FROM ARTHRITIS

Whenever arthritis prevents full range of movement of the back or any joint, and whenever bed rest is required, deformities of the joints may result, and permanent restricting of movement can occur.

To prevent the stiffness and deformities as much as possible, here are the guidelines given to us by the doctors we interviewed.

• Don't rest for long periods with your knees flexed. For example, don't put pillows under your knees when resting in bed, but keep the legs extended.

• Don't sit for a prolonged time in a chair or rest for a long time on a soft bed. The bed should be firm and you should get up occasionally and move about.

• Don't use a thick pillow if there is upper spine or neck arthritis. Keep the spine in as normal a position as possible when in bed.

• Do therapeutic exercises designed to maintain the range of motion of the joints at least once, preferably twice, a day.

Special warning: Don't immobilize an inflamed joint or a joint affected with osteoarthritis for prolonged periods. When a joint is immobilized, the cartilage undergoes very rapid defective changes, according to a recent warning by Dr. Marshall Palmoski and Dr. Kenneth Brandt, of the University of Indiana Medical

Center. They say that cartilage is not the inert tissue it was long believed to be. For example, even in teen-age patients, who have not used their joints or borne weight on them for prolonged periods, the doctors found the cartilage tissues "were a complete mess," with changes just like those of osteoarthritis. In fact, the doctors said, some cartilage changes that until now have been attributed to osteoarthritis may actually result from lack of weight-bearing and/or lack of usage.

NEW TREATMENTS

Folic acid pills. Significant success in improving joint mobility and eliminating pain has been described by a number of doctors. Some doctors use 1-milligram tablets; others as much as 5 milligrams per day. In the United States a prescription is needed for 1-milligram tablets of this vitamin; in Canada 5-milligram tablets can be bought over the counter in any drugstore.

Copper aspirinate. This copper-aspirin combination eliminates the bad side effects of aspirin, guarding against ulcers, and in clinical tests appears to be some twenty times more effective than plain aspirin, and five to eight times more effective than cortisone.

Zinc sulfate. At the University of Washington, patients with chronic rheumatoid arthritis who were given zinc sulfate tablets three times daily had less joint tenderness, swelling, and stiffness. "These encouraging results," says investigator Peter S. Simkin, "indicate that oral zinc sulfate deserves further study in patients with active rheumatoid arthritis." Other researchers recommend a zinc complex tablet, saying it is absorbed better and causes less gastrointestinal difficulty.

Gold pills. These new pills are faster and more effective than ordinary injections of gold, say developers at Smith, Kline and French Laboratories. The pills, called Auranofin, are being further tested now in Argentina, Sweden, and South Africa. The pills are reported to take effect in about five weeks (injections take about three months) with dramatic reducing of joint pain, swelling, and stiffness.

A new drug to stop aspirin damage. A hormone called prostaglandin E₂ has been shown to prevent the damage to the digestive system often caused by aspirin and indomethacin. Dr. Max Cohen said at a meeting of the American College of Surgeons that prostaglandin works by increasing the protection of the digestive system against acid.

Radiotherapy. This is frequently used to treat the active phase of ankylosing spondylitis. In early cases the results are excellent, and the disease process is apparently arrested.

DMSO. Short for dimethyl sulfoxide, DMSO, as discussed earlier, has been shown to reduce pain and increase joint mobility in many persons with osteoarthritis.

Orgotein. This new anti-inflammatory drug is being studied in eleven major medical centers in the United States and various other countries. It has an outstanding safety record in the trials of its use for arthritis, cataracts, and inflammations of the genitourinary tract. Investigators are very enthusiastic about its benefits. Orgotein is already available to practicing physicians in Austria, and is available in the United States from Diagnostic Data, Inc., in California, but only to veterinarians to treat dogs and horses. The new drug contains an enzyme called superoxide dismutase found naturally in the body, and appears to be particularly effective for rheumatoid arthritis and osteoarthritis. Safety tests are excellent, with no side effects being reported in more than 600,000 injections. The drug has also been used to counteract radiation side effects in cancer patients. In animals it is approved for the relief of inflammation associated with ankylosing spondylitis, spondylosis, and disk disease.

Sulindac. This new drug has been shown to be effective in the treatment of most kinds of arthritis, including rheumatoid arthritis, osteoarthritis, gouty arthritis, and ankylosing spondylitis. For several years it has been available for investigational use only in the United States, but has now just been released for general use. It is long-lasting (only two pills a day are needed) and is less irritating to the stomach than aspirin. (It is also helpful in bursitis of the shoulder.) It is about as effective as eight aspirin per day.

Penicillamine. This medicine is at present approved in the United States only for investigation to treat arthritis. It appears comparable to gold in providing slow but long-term benefits in some patients, and helps many people with rheumatoid arthritis in whom gold does not work. The drug is currently being tested simultaneously in the United States in eleven major medical centers and in the USSR on a cooperative basis. It has been approved and has been used successfuly in the past to treat Wilson's disease, a rare illness of the liver and the nervous system, as well as to eliminate lead from the body. Reports from France show about 80 percent of patients respond, but many people have to stop the drug because of the side effects. The most common penicillamine side effect is skin rash, but serious blood and kidney disorders can also occur. Patients should take the medication only if they do not respond to other treatment, and they should have frequent blood and urine tests to monitor for possible trouble.

Rheumanx. This controversial remedy for arthritis, developed by doctors in Canada, is about to become available in several countries. The key ingredients are prednisone, testosterone, and estradiol, compounded together and claimed by the developers to be helpful in many cases of rheumatoid arthritis, gout, osteoarthritis, and ankylosing spondylitis. Clinics using the formula are presently operating in the Dominican Republic, Mexico, and Canada. The substance will soon be available in England to physicians who may order it from Switzerland for use in specific patients.

Spare parts. When joints are badly destroyed by arthritis, sometimes replacement with an artificial joint is the most satisfactory answer. An artificial joint for the hip is now widely used (80,000 were implanted last year) and is dramatically effective. Early results in replacement of shoulder joints are encouraging also. Contact local chapters of the Arthritis Foundation for recommended surgeons nearest you who do the operation you might need.

A new kind of surgery for hips. A new technique of resurfacing the hip joint may soon be available to patients who do not need total hip joint replacement. Dr. Chitranjan Ranawat, of the Hospital for Special Surgery in New York City, explains that when the entire hip joint is replaced, the head of the femur (leg bone) is sawed off and replaced by a metal ball with a long stem, which is cemented into the femur. A polyethylene cup is cemented into the pelvic bone. With the new operation, the head of the femur is simply capped with a metal covering, and the pelvic cup is cleaned and lined with polyethylene. Pain relief and functional improvement of the simple resurfacing operation are comparable to traditional surgery, and the threat of infection is reduced, the doctor says.

Oiling the joints. Doctors at the Institute of Experimental and Clinical Medicine in Lithuania have found that artificial lubrication is helpful to osteoarthritis patients with aching joints. They reported at an International Congress of Rheumatology meeting that a synthetic type of joint fluid (made of a chemical called polyvinylpyrrolidine) injected into the joints weekly for four to six weeks brought improvement to patients with osteoarthritis of the knee, hip, and shoulder joints. Function improved, pain lessened or disappeared, and mobility increased. The good results have been confirmed in Japanese studies, where a natural enzyme called hyaluronic acid was also added to the injection mixture.

ARTHRITIS EXERCISES

The following exercises are recommended by the Arthritis Foundation for strengthening and stretching muscles, increasing the range of motion of joints, and improving function.

Stand with your back against a wall and your buttocks, shoulder blades, and head touching it. Grasp a broomstick or cane in both hands and raise it as high above your head as possible, keeping your elbows as straight as you can. Then lower your arms. Repeat.

Grab the stick and push it up as if you were shoveling snow over your right shoulder. Change your grip and repeat the motion over your left shoulder. Repeat.

The Foundation also recommends a Single Knee Raise (Better Back Exercise 6).

Do the arthritis exercises at least twice per day, the Foundation suggests. Start gently and slowly, gradually trying to increase joint function. Some pain during exercise is normal, but if it persists the next day, you have overdone it and should cut back. When joints are inflamed in an acute attack, do not do the exercises.

POSTURE WHEN YOU HAVE ARTHRITIS

The first instinct of every person with arthritis is to find a position that is most comfortable for a painful joint, and then keep the joint in that position for long periods. Usually that position is one in which the joint is bent to some degree. Comfortable or not, this is the worst thing you can do, says the Arthritis Foundation. It leads to greater stiffness and loss of joint mobility and, eventually, to deformity.

Posture Checklist

Standing   Stand straight, head high, shoulders straight, stomach in, hips and knees straight.

Walking   Walk erect, as in standing position.
Keep your hips and knees straight.
Let your arms swing easily at your sides.
Do not sag or shuffle.

Sitting   Use a straight-back arm chair with a firm seat.
Sit with your head up, shoulders straight, stomach in.
Keep your feet flat on the floor.

In bed   Lie straight, flat on your back.
Keep your knees and hips straight, arms and hands straight at your sides.
Use a board between the mattress and bedspring to keep the mattress firm.
If you need a pillow under your head, use a small one.
Never put a pillow under your knees.

FLUOROSIS (Also called Osteofluorosis)

Few members of the public or even of the medical profession know that one crippling form of arthritis can be caused by overexposure to fluorides. Progressive stiffness, pain, and limitation of motion occur in the back and resemble ankylosing spondylitis or severe rickets. Crippling from fluorosis occurs frequently in certain areas of the world like India and Africa, where there is a combination of a high content of fluoride in the water (four parts per million) and a high consumption of water because of the hot, dry climate. It also occurs in some areas where there is a high intake of tea or of foods grown in soil with a high fluoride content. The disease is relatively rare in the United States, but may occur in persons who drink a lot of water.

Excess fluoride is deposited in the bones and often produces bony projections and growths. At first, the neck becomes stiff, then the back, with possible formation of a hump. Ligaments and joints become hardened. The spine may become rigid and the vertebrae sometimes become fused. Usually it takes some twenty years of exposure before such symptoms appear, but if exposure is extreme, the disease can occur in childern.

GOUT OF THE SPINE

A big toe is the usual spot that gout attacks, but it can also occur in the spine or hip joint. The cause—the same as gout of other joints—is a deposit of urate crystals in the joint; the involved joint then becomes very tender. Spine or hip involvement may occur with an attack of the big toe, or separately.

Diagnosis. High levels of uric acid in the blood, and chalky stonelike deposits of urate crystals that can be detected by X-ray or clinical examination.

Treatment. The same gout medicines used for other forms of gout, such as colchicine. Sometimes indomethacin or phenyl-butazone are helpful in controlling or lessening attacks. For chronic conditions, a diet eliminating internal organs such as kidneys or liver that contain high levels of uric acid should be followed to reduce uric acid levels in the blood that, by precipitating out, cause the problems in the joints.

HELPFUL RESOURCES FOR ARTHRITIS PATIENTS

Accent on Living. Magazine for people with disabilities. Box 700, Bloomington, Illinois 61701.

Self-Help Devices. Descriptions, sources, prices of hundreds of devices. 193 pages. Institute of Rehabilitation Medicine, New York University Medical Center, 400 E. 34th St., New York, New York 10016. $4.

Toomey Gazette. Suggestions for dealing with disabilities. Box 147, Chagrin Falls, Ohio 44022.

Handbooks on *Rheumatoid Arthritis, Osteoarthritis* and *Gout.* All free. The Arthritis Foundation, 3400 Peachtree St. NE, Atlanta, Georgia 30326.

Rehabilitation Gazette. 4502 Maryland Avenue, St. Louis, Missouri 63108. $2.

Arthritis Information Clearinghouse. National Institute of Arthritis, Metabolism and Digestive Diseases, Bethesda, Maryland 20014. Educational materials for physicians and patients available.

DIET AND ARTHRITIS

The Arthritis Foundation says unequivocably that there is no relationship between arthritis and diet, but there is heated controversy over this among some doctors. As one doctor, who refused to be quoted, said: "I agree that calcium, for example, does not miraculously cure arthritis, but I believe what is often called arthritis pain really isn't. The pain is caused or aggravated by demineralization of bones, and calcium does help that."

Many patients who were on painkilling drugs daily with what they thought was arthritis say they have found relief with bone meal or other calcium supplementation, some being free from pain for years, even though pain was so severe they were scheduled for total hip replacement.

An article in the *British Medical Journal* points out that many patients with advanced arthritis rarely leave the house and so do not receive much vitamin D from sunlight, which may play an important role in the bone frailty of patients with longstanding arthritis. The authors recommend daily supplements of vitamin D.

A Rutgers University scientist, Dr. Norman F. Childers, a horticulturist of New Brunswick, New Jersey, and author of *Nightshades and Health,* claims that the nightshade group of plants can cause arthritis symptoms in many people. If persons are sensitive to them, they can have a full-blown arthritis attack by eating foods in this family, Dr. Childers says. He has case histories of more than 2,000 people who claim to have had great relief from pain when they excluded from their diets such foods as white potatoes, peppers, paprika, eggplant, and tomato. Patients' symptoms returned if they allowed the foods back in their diet. Dr. Childers does not say that all people suffering from arthritis should avoid these foods, but that *some* patients are sensitive to them, as well as to tobacco, which is in the nightshade family. Dr. Childers notes that it may require at least three months of complete abstinence from these foods (and preferably tobacco) before benefits can be noticed.

A number of doctors report success with vitamin B supplements to help alleviate the symptoms of rheumatoid arthritis. They have found folic acid, one of the B relatives, to be particularly helpful. Dr. William Kaufman reports in the *Journal of the*

American Geriatrics Association that, in 663 patients, he found that large doses of the B vitamin niacinamide increased joint mobility without exception in every patient. Not all patients improved equally well, and not all joints improved equally, but every person reported an improvement of some kind, he said.

The late Dr. John J. Miller, founder of Miller Pharmacal Company, felt strongly that large doses of vitamins and minerals were beneficial in arthritis and osteoporosis. He gathered together evidence from research literature that one could help prevent tissue degeneration by taking magnesium, calcium, and vitamins D and E. He also cited evidence that lubrication in the joints and strength and elasticity of connective tissues were helped by taking magnesium, zinc, vitamins A, D, C, and E, bioflavinoids, vitamin B12, paraaminobenzoic acid (PABA) and pantothenate, both vitamin B relatives. He recommended that patients take supplements of all these vitamins and minerals and test for themselves whether they benefited by the change.

At the risk of being redundant, there is one thing about which there is no controversy—one of the best diet moves you can make for arthritis is to get rid of excess weight. This will take the extra strain off your body and will also make increased exercise possible, which, in turn, will increase general fitness and bone density.

26 What to Do for a Slipped Disk

A spinal disk is the cushionlike pad that separates all the vertebrae and helps absorb the shocks of everyday activity to your spine. Disks are made of tough, fibrous cartilage packed with water and a protein called "ground substance." They are a valuable and necessary functional part of the back.

Trouble can start when there is a sudden injury that causes the disk to rupture or when there is long-term stress and strain or when degenerative changes occur over the years. There may be immediate, sudden, complete rupture or bulging, or the slippage may be gradual and progressive. The disk may rupture or slip backward or to one side. Pain may be racking and sudden, or may be intermittent, occurring with certain positions or during certain activities. Whether the doctor calls it herniated disk, slipped disk, ruptured disk, sliding disk, protruding disk, disk syndrome, or ruptured nucleus pulposus, the mechanism of pain is the same—the tough disk bulges or slips out of its normal position and pushes against sensitive nerve fibers as they course into the spinal cord, causing pain. If the disk pushes against the sciatic nerve coming from the hip and legs, it causes the pain called sciatica.

Most doctors consider derangements of the disks the most overwhelmingly common cause of back pain. One doctor said at least half of the adult population can expect to be incapacitated with low back pain due to disk disease at some time in their lives. One study showed herniated disk was most likely to be found among persons aged thirty to thirty-nine, and that the most important risk factors among the variables considered in this study were driving motor vehicles and sedentary occupations. Other doctors point out that "slipped disk" is much more frequently blamed for back pain in the United States than in other countries, is often incorrectly blamed for back pain, and that frequently patients are operated on for this ailment when it doesn't even exist.

One doctor told me that many persons who think they are suffering from disk trouble actually are victims of strain of the back muscles.

Back pain from disk degeneration most often begins with mild back pain. The patient recalls that after periods of prolonged physical activity or working in a position that causes stress to the spine, pain appears in the lower back. The pain usually lasts only a few days and subsides with limitation of activity and bed rest. The pain is made worse by standing and lifting and is relieved by rest. This on-again off-again pain is characteristic of disk disease. With the passage of time, the episodes may become more frequent and more intense and lead to more disability. A trivial accident, such as bending forward to shave, coughing, or stooping to pick up an object from the floor, may precipitate a severe attack. (Pain that is unrelenting and progressive and that is worse when the patient is in bed at night is more suggestive of cancer.)

Most disk pain occurs in the lower back, but degeneration of disks of the vertebrae of the neck and thoracic area can also cause pain in the neck and upper back.

HOW DO YOU KNOW IF YOU HAVE A DISK PROBLEM?

The following signs point to disk syndrome:
A history of injury or repeated strains to the back.
Back pain followed by leg pain.
Loss of sense of touch in some areas of the back or legs.
Lowered skin temperature over the top of the foot.
Weakness of some muscles, especially in thigh or calf or big toe.
Diminished knee jerk or ankle jerk reflexes.
Leg pain produced or increased by coughing, sneezing, or bearing-down abdominal pressure, as in defecation.
Treatment actually becomes the final diagnosis, says Dr.

Richard Leedy of Woodbury, New Jersey. If the condition is just a back sprain, he reports, then relaxation of the muscle spasm by a local anesthetic such as lidocaine plus manipulative therapy to stretch the muscles and restore balance and motion between the joints produce dramatic relief of pain. If pain is not relieved, then disk syndrome should be strongly considered.

The Straight Leg Test

Lie down on the floor with your legs stretched straight out. Have someone raise one leg. If the leg will not raise straight up to the normal 90 degrees or if pain is produced in *either* leg, there is a 95 percent chance that disk syndrome is present. If when the ankle is bent by pushing the toes toward the head, thus stretching the sciatic nerve even farther, the pain becomes worse or produces pain at a lower level, it is even further confirmation of disk trouble, although there is still some chance the problem may be muscle spasm.

X-rays do not help much in diagnosis, but your doctor may take X-rays to find any changes in the spine that have occurred. (Simple thinning of the disk space does not necessarily indicate disk syndrome.)

Other aids to diagnosis. Electromyography, myelography, and discography, although these last two are usually not done unless surgery is being seriously considered, since they are not simple tests to do.

WHAT TO DO WHEN YOU HAVE AN ACUTE ATTACK

Rest in bed with only bathroom privileges.

While in bed, keep hips and knees flexed to a comfortable degree.

Don't sleep face down.

Use a natural or synthetic sheepskin to provide comfort with prolonged bed rest.

Only in the horizontal position is the disk free of significant stress. Sitting at a desk or in an armchair does not provide adequate relief from stress.

If the disk attack is severe, some doctors believe one or two weeks of complete bed rest may be required, whether at home or in the hospital, then a week to ten days of gradual mobilization if there has been substantial relief of pain. Other doctors feel bed rest should be for only a short time because of the loss of muscle tone, weakening, and depression that can occur.

Your physician may give you an anti-inflammatory drug such as phenylbutazone (Butazolidin), a muscle relaxant such as methocarbamol (Robaxin) or carisoprodal (Soma) if there is muscle spasm, and a pain reliever such as aspirin or codeine or morphine if necessary.

Some doctors give a sedative or mild tranquilizer, which does not help the back, but does alleviate anxiety and make the prolonged period of bed rest more tolerable.

Some physicians reported that vitamin B supplements were helpful since they strengthen and apparently help the irritated nerve tissue that is causing pain.

Some physicians say application of heat is helpful; others feel that, although it may give temporary relief, it can result in increased muscle spasm later.

Most doctors we talked to felt traction was not helpful for disk problems in the neck. If traction is used, the patient should be hospitalized and have complete bed rest.

A rigid lumbar brace is seldom recommended, since victims are better off with a program designed to increase the range of motion and strengthen musculature. (Sometimes, however, braces or corsets are used for support in elderly patients or in obese patients with poor abdominal musculature until they develop their abdominal muscles and lose weight.)

Some doctors feel gentle manipulation is very helpful, often aiding patients who have not been helped by anything else; others feel it could cause nerve damage.

Sprays of ethyl chloride or similar coolants are of value in reducing pain and muscle spasm.

Muscle spasms can also be reduced by a soft tissue massage, massaging along muscle lines of the body and pushing away from the spine.

If there is any question concerning the diagnosis, consultation with another doctor is indicated since there are many conditions that mimic the herniated disk syndrome.

After two to three weeks, when symptoms have mostly subsided, nearly every doctor we talked to strongly recommended the patient begin back exercises like those we have outlined in the Better Back Ten-Week Exercise Program. Start the exercises slowly and gently, and discontinue them immediately if a flare-up of symptoms appears. They may be reinstituted at a later date when tolerance has increased.

IF YOU HAVE A MANIPULATION

Dr. Charles Steiner, osteopathic physician of Piscataway, New Jersey, gives this advice to patients. After treatment, perform a few knee-bending exercises while holding on to a counter or to a tabletop with both hands. The motion is helpful in rotating the pelvis forward and convinces a frightened patient that his or her legs can support the body. Repeat this exercise at least four times daily.

Also, he says, take a warm bath before retiring to achieve body relaxation, sinking deep into the tub so that your shoulders are under the water.

Motion should be encouraged. Avoid any posture that fosters a freezing of the muscles and joints into any one position.

HOW TO TELL IF IMPROVEMENT IS LIKELY TO LAST

Simple conservative measures help many cases of herniated disk, and manipulation has been shown to give good results in about 60 percent of patients. But how do you know if, after several months, clinical improvement will continue, or whether symptoms will get worse or begin to come back again?

One test, physicians say, is electromyography, a technique of measuring the electric charges of muscle fibers served by individual nerves. By analyzing the action potential produced on an oscilloscope, doctors can tell whether there is definite compression and squeezing of the nerve by the out-of-place disk at the spinal cord.

If there is no electromyographic evidence of nerve root compression, there probably will be improvement from manipulation, and the improvement will probably last. When there is electromyographic evidence of nerve root compression, there may be temporary clinical improvement, but it probably will not last and more radical treatment probably will be needed.

SCIATICA

The sciatic nerve comes from the spinal cord, goes to and along the back muscles, and also supplies the muscles and skin of the legs and feet. If there is pressure or tension on the nerve where it emerges from the spinal cord, there can be severe pain all along the course of the nerve. The pressure can be from something as simple as muscle imbalance and muscle tension, or it can be from an infection or an injury, or it can be caused by pressure or pinching from a tumor, or—usually the case—a slipped spinal disk.

There may be a deep ache or a sharp, stabbing pain that runs down the back of the buttocks and hip to the thigh or below the mid-calf of the leg. Usually there is stiffness in forward bending, although sideways bending is effortless. The degree of pain may vary from strong discomfort to such severity that the patient cannot stand or walk. A sneeze or cough or any sudden jolt of the spine can cause searing pain.

About 35 percent of people complaining of low back pain eventually develop sciatica if they do not take adequate measures to strengthen their backs.

Tests for Sciatica

Test 1. Sit on the edge of a table with both legs dangling, back as erect as possible and arms hanging at the sides. Have someone place a hand firmly on your thigh just above the knee. Have them put their other hand under the heel of the same leg, and gradually straighten the leg by pushing the heel upward. They should keep raising the leg upward higher than the point of being level. If there is no tension or sciatica, the leg should straighten out with no resistance or discomfort. If you tend to flip over backward or have to brace yourself with your hands to keep from falling back, sciatic nerve tension is indicated. Test one leg, then the other.

Test 2. Lie on your back on a table or floor, with your legs outstretched, toes pointed. Have someone place a hand under the heel of your foot and gradually raise the leg, keeping it fully extended. If your knee automatically buckles and the leg bends when it is raised about halfway, sciatic nerve tension is present. Test one leg, then the other.

Test 3. Sit on the floor or table with both legs together extended straight out in front. If you can sit with your back straight and without leaning on your arms for support, there probably is no sciatic tension. If you need to support yourself, or bend your knees or curve your back, it indicates that there probably is sciatic tension.

Other signs. Pain is aggravated when you twist the body, is worse when sitting, and is sometimes relieved by standing up or lying flat.

What to Do for Sciatica

The pain will often disappear by itself in a few weeks or months.

Bed rest is usually recommended as the best treatment. (Lie on your back with a pillow under the lower back and the knees; use a firm mattress or bedboard.) However, there is some argument over this. A doctor writing in a Danish medical journal, *Ugeskrift for Laeger,* reported on two sets of sciatica patients, 100 treated by complete bed rest, the other attempting normal movement as soon as possible. The bed-rest patients remained in the hospital an average of fifty days, the others for thirty days. Most doctors we asked said stay in bed till the pain lessens enough so that you feel like getting up (up to fourteen days for severe sciatica).

See your doctor for pain-relieving drugs and a muscle relaxant drug.

A hot bath or heating pad will occasionally give relief.

Exercising in bed is sometimes helpful, lifting your legs and moving them from side to side.

Manipulation is often helpful.

Injections of Novocain or other drugs may be given to block nerve impulses.

Vitamins may be given orally or by injection. Injections of vitamin B1 were reported successful in relieving pain of sciatica.

Traction (stretching the leg by attaching weights) may be necessary. Ultrasound, diathermy, and whirlpool boths are sometimes helpful.

Surgery should be postponed and used only as a last resort.

After an attack. Wearing a corset to restrict back movement is often recommended. No heavy work should be done without the approval of your doctor. Check with your doctor as to whether you have a calcium or vitamin B deficiency and should take supplements to help prevent future attacks.

Note: Sciatica pain can also be produced by cancer of the prostate and by diabetic nerve degeneration.

Leg pain resembling sciatica can often be caused by flat feet. If you think this could be your problem, try this exercise. Stand with both feet on a rolling pin. Hold on to something to steady yourself and roll back and forth, as far backward and as far forward as possible. Do 6 to 10 times. This lifts the bones of the arch and releases pressure on the nerve that causes the leg pain. Do not walk around after the exercise, but keep weight off your feet.

SHOULD YOU HAVE SURGERY?

About 20 percent of patients with a firm diagnosis of disk lesion ultimately will require surgery at some point. Most doctors interviewed said they never consider surgery for a disk problem until the patient has tried conservative treatment for at least two months. The only reason they would perform surgery earlier is if the patient had unbearably severe pain or if there are symptoms of actual nerve damage, such as bladder or bowel disturbances, or paralysis of any muscles.

On the other hand, doctors said, if you have diligently followed an exercise program and other instructions for two months and still have severe pain, do not put off surgery if your doctor recommends it, because delay then is of no benefit.

One word of caution: Discuss in detail with your doctor how much pain relief he expects you might have. Sometimes surgery will give complete relief; in other cases, patients can only expect relief of leg pain, not back pain. Most patients who have surgery still have occasional back trouble if they do not follow up with a sustained exercise program like the one we have outlined in this book.

As one doctor said, "Too many operations for low back pain have been performed. The two most common surgical procedures are laminectomies and spinal fusions (joining two or more vertebrae). Although 200,000 of these operations are done annually, up to 40 percent of them fail to achieve the desired results." The mortality rate is low for surgery (1 per 3,000), he says, but the other risks are considerable. Often the scar tissue that forms as a result of the surgery actually increases pain.

Dr. Anders Hakelius, of Karolinska Institut in Copenhagen, did a comparative study of patients with disk problems who were operated on or were treated only conservatively without surgery for their back pain and sciatica. Patients ranged in age from nine to sixty-seven, but were mostly in the thirty to forty-nine age bracket. Follow-up examinations were done after seven years. Of those operated on, more were free of symptoms *during* the seven years and had fewer recurrences of back pain attacks than those who did not have surgery. But at the *end* of the seven years, both groups were the same in terms of pain and number of attacks.

One doctor estimated that, in his experience, after removal of a disk only about 15 percent of those operated on obtained complete and permanent relief of their pain. And fusing the two vertebrae together after removal of the disk, he said, doesn't guarantee permanent relief either and may place added stress on the adjacent disks.

Most doctors said that unless there is a possibility of a tumor, a fracture, or irreversible anatomic defect, the results of conservative treatment usually are equally as good as surgical treatment. Patients for whom surgery has been recommended should always ask for a second opinion if the surgeon cannot predict a better outcome than what would result from a nonsurgical approach. In the final analysis, surgery isn't necessary for most types of back pain.

The patient and doctor must make the decision together. In general, surgery is recommended only after careful diagnostic evaluation—when a firm diagnosis is established, a concerted course of conservative treatment has failed, and the attending surgeon believes with certainty that operative intervention would alleviate the disease process.

THE ENZYME TREATMENT THAT SOME SAY COULD ALMOST MAKE BACK SURGERY UNNECESSARY

Chymopapain, an enzyme derived from the papaya plant and often used as a meat tenderizer, has now moved from the kitchen to the operating room. It is being used to dissolve slipped, sliding, ruptured, or protruding spinal disks, making it possible for thousands of patients to avoid the back surgery that formerly would have been the only treatment for their unbearable pain.

The enzyme is injected into the disk where it breaks down the protein within the disk so the protein and stored water can escape and be absorbed into the body. The disk, minus the bulging water and protein, slips back into place between the vertebrae, eliminating the pressure on the nerves that was causing the pain.

Doctors using chymopapain report excellent results. So far about three out of four patients treated have complete relief of pain. It works best on young patients with badly herniated disks or severe sciatica that has not responded to traditional treatment.

Since about 1 out of 100 people has an allergic reaction to the enzyme, it is injected in the hospital under general anesthesia so any reactions can be dealt with easily and promptly.

The medical name for the technique is chemonucleolysis. It involves no scalpel, no blood—just injection of the enzyme via a long needle inserted into the patient's back. Proper placement is assured by careful monitoring of the insertion using X-ray and television. The needles are left in for about five minutes.

The developer of the technique, Dr. Lyman Smith, surgeon at Northwestern University in Chicago, has treated more than 10,000 patients this way. The main advantage, he says, is that the patient can avoid the prolonged bed rest that often accompanies traditional back surgery.

Many doctors feel the injection technique should be tried before surgery is considered for any patients, since surgery with its attendant possible risks and complications always can be tried later if injection does not work. In fact, they say it is *the* treatment of choice if standard conservative treatments have failed.

Dr. David Teperson, orthopedic surgeon of Hollywood, Florida, reports a typical case. A forty-two-year-old insurance adjuster and riding enthusiast was racked with excruciating pain one day. A herniated disk was diagnosed by several doctors, and surgery was recommended. The patient had heard of the injections, however, and requested that procedure. Three long needles were inserted and the enzyme was injected. The entire process lasted less than thirty minutes. Five days later she left the hospital, in four weeks was back at work, had no pain, and could even ride her horse again. (Some patients need several weeks to recover, but none require the long recovery time they would following surgery.)

The enzyme technique can also be used on patients who have had previous back surgery that has not been successful, often bringing about relief for the first time after years of terrible pain.

The enzyme is used *only* for treating disk problems. It will not work for back pain due to arthritis, pulled muscles, tension, or other causes.

Despite its success rate, the technique is still very controversial. Its history has been strange. In 1941 the enzyme was isolated from the papaya tree. Experiments on animals indicated its medical promise, and in 1964 Dr. Lyman Smith and his associates showed what it could do in the treatment of disk problems in humans. Other doctors began to try the enzyme treatment and were enthusiastic. Travenol Laboratories manufactured the enzyme preparation under the name Discase. By 1974 more than 10,000 patients had been treated, with good results. By 1975 some 1,600 physicians had been trained to use the enzyme and were awaiting its approval by the Food and Drug Administration. The FDA Surgical Drugs Advisory Committee had recommended the drug's release, and approval was promised by the director of Surgical–Dental Products of the FDA. Then suddenly, in July, 1975, all investigators were ordered by registered letter to give no further injections as of that moment and to return all supplies on hand because a new double-blind study of the enzyme was going to be done in four medical centers—San Francisco V.A. Hospital, University of Minnesota Medical Center, Walter Reed Army Medical Center, and the University of Miami School of Medicine. ("Double blind" meant it would be compared to another substance and no one would know which patients got which treatments.)

In November, 1975, the results of the double-blind study were presented to a meeting of officers of the American Academy of Orthopedic Surgeons, FDA officials, and Travenol Laboratories representatives. It was reported that the control injections, containing a substance called EDTA, used for comparison, appeared to have some therapeutic benefit of its own and that Discase was only 10 percent better than the control. Some representatives at the meeting recommended that chymopapain be withdrawn from further investigative use; others recommended a release that would allow physicians, instructed in its use, to administer the enzyme under a certain protocol that also required they report any adverse reactions. No action was ever taken by the FDA. The new drug application for Discase was withdrawn. And that's where things still sit. Meanwhile, patients who are candidates for chemonucleolysis must go to Canada or England where the enzyme treatment is available and where doctors continue to report good results.

Many doctors were upset and frustrated. Dr. Mark D. Brown and Dr. Robert B. Daroff, of the University of Miami, Florida, who were themselves participants in the FDA's double-blind study, decried the decision and challenged the conclusions reached from the study's data. Results on patients were analyzed too soon, they said, being recorded less than six weeks after injection, before results could validly be compared; the doses of Discase allowed in the study were lower than surgeons recommended, and the EDTA used as a control actually did have some benefit and so was not a real control.

To add to the controversy, there seems to be a split between specialties. Orthopedic surgeons tend to think the enzyme treatment should be tried on patients who have failed to respond to conservative treatment before they are subjected to surgery. Neurosurgeons report they have heard the enzyme treatment can cause complications, even paralysis.

Just as this book went to press, a new study was authorized by the FDA for Travenol Laboratories to use larger doses and for longer times before evaluation. That study is now underway.

What results have there actually been with the enzyme? Dr. Brown reports that of his patients, all candidates for surgery, 70 percent had satisfactory relief of symptoms and returned to previous employment. No patient was made worse, and patients were out of the hospital and back to work quickly, a huge savings when compared to convalescence needed following disk surgery. Chemonucleolysis is also safer, he said.

Dr. Eugene S. Nordby, of the University of Wisconsin School of Medicine, compared a group of patients treated by surgery and a group treated with the enzyme, all of whom were problem patients in severe pain prior to treatment. Of the patients treated with the enzyme, 74 percent had good or excellent results; and of the patients having surgery, only 48 percent had good or excellent results. And two patients having surgery got worse, he said.

Enzyme-treated patients had less postoperative pain. The average time needed to return to work was 66 days, compared to 202 days for those having surgery. "Economic implications of being off work, whether or not one is receiving Workmen's Compensation payments, is obvious and to our minds impressive," Nordby says. He believes the enzyme treatment would spare at least 75 percent of disk patients destined for surgery. "The drug should be reapproved for investigational use," he says.

Dr. Burton Onofrio, of the Mayo Clinic, found chemonucleolysis or laminectomy patients had good results.

Drs. Leon Wiltse, Eric Weidell, Jr., and Hansen A. Yaun, of Long Beach, California, reported on 500 patients treated by chemonucleolysis and concluded that the results were as good as with a laminectomy . . . 75 percent had effective relief of symptoms. It was Wiltse who successfully did chemonucleolysis on Chicago White Sox third baseman Bill Melton for his herniated disk.

Dr. Eugene Dabezies and Dr. Michael Brunet, of Louisiana State University, report 71 percent of enzyme-treated patients had good to excellent recovery, compared to 63 percent of surgery patients. They too believe it could potentially eliminate three fourths of back operations in the United States.

The clinical experience of forty-five surgeons in 10,000 cases over ten years indicates that 70 percent of patients show marked improvement following enzyme treatment, 14 percent slight improvement, and 16 percent no improvement. Improvement statistics are not as good if patients had previous surgery.

Meanwhile, hundreds of American citizens are traveling to Canada to be treated with the enzyme. Many United States doctors still believe the enzyme is of no benefit, but others think it's great and are referring their patients to medical centers in Canada—and sometimes go themselves. For example, a Chicago orthopedic surgeon sent twenty to twenty-five patients to Canada—then needed help himself. He referred himself to Toronto's Wellesley Hospital and was injected with chymopapain last year. He says his back troubles have disappeared.

You should not have the enzyme treatment if you are allergic to meat tenderizer, papaya, or beer because of the increased likelihood of allergic reaction to the enzyme.

FACET DENERVATION—IT MAY BE EVEN BETTER

This is a technique that may prove to be better than either surgery or enzyme treatment.

A facet is one of the little flat surfaces on the vertebrae of the spinal cord where the joints come together. Tiny nerve roots come into the spinal cord there. The newest technique that looks promising is one that destroys these tiny nerve branches to the facets by electrocoagulation through a needle. This newest approach is called facet rhizotomy or facet denervation.

One developer of the technique, Dr. C. Norman Shealy, director of the Pain and Health Rehabilitation Center, of La Crosse, Wisconsin, says the majority of patients diagnosed as having slipped or herniated disks are wrongly diagnosed and really have disturbances in these facet joints and the nerve branches near them.

Dr. Shealy believes that for most patients, even those with severe back pain, all conservative treatments, including bed rest, painkillers, external electrical stimulation, ice packs, acupuncture, nerve block injections, biofeedback, and exercises, should be tried before considering facet denervation. But he advises, the technique should be considered seriously in all patients before a disk operation is done, because facet denervation is safer and simpler. It is even safer than chemonucleolysis with papaya enzyme, he says, and results are superior. No neurological complications have been reported in 800 patients surveyed so far.

In undergoing facet denervation, the patient is placed face down on a fluoroscope table, awake so he or she can discuss any sensations with the surgeon, and the procedure is followed by X-ray. A thin needle is introduced through the skin and muscle to touch the facets of one or more vertebrae. When properly situated, a probe is advanced through the needle, and the needle itself is removed. After further adjustment, the nerve is electrically stimulated, and the patient tells the doctor if his pain is like the original pain and is reproduced in the same area. If so, then the nerve is coagulated with a burst of radiofrequency and the electrode is removed. No surgical cutting is necessary. The patient is immediately forced to walk and begins limbering exercises.

In 380 patients treated at La Crosse, Dr. Shealy reports 82 percent of those with low back pain benefited "significantly," unless they had had previous disk removal or fusion, in which case benefits were fewer.

Dr. William Finney and Dr. D. Graham Slaughter, of Baltimore, treated 270 patients and reported about 80 percent excellent or good results in those who had not had previous disk surgery. (Only 50 to 60 percent of patients with previous surgery were helped.) Several hundred other surgeons are now also using the technique, with similar benefits.

"These results suggest the necessity for a major reappraisal of our surgical approach to the disk syndrome," says Shealy. The truth is, he says, that most patients do not do well with the now "traditional" approach of disk removal, so this new procedure should play a major role in effectively relieving pain in the future in most back problems. "Before resorting to laminectomy, or to either myelography of discography, we recommend consideration of radiofrequency facet denervation," he says. "The procedure has an amazingly benign record and an excellent chance of accomplishing satisfactory pain relief."

Actually, Dr. Shealy believes ruptured disk is very rare, occurring in less than 1 percent of people with back trouble. A diagnosis of ruptured disk is usually a false one, he told us, and the pain is usually caused by other things, such as muscle strain or abnormalities of the joint capsule of the vertebrae.

Most of the disk surgery now performed can be avoided by the new facet denervation technique, Shealy says, saving time, money, and surgical risk, and providing better pain relief.

27 When Your Bones Get Weak— Osteoporosis

Osteoporosis is probably the most common disease of the bones encountered in the doctor's clinical practice. In this disorder, the bone becomes less dense and the amount of bone in the body—the total bone mass—decreases.

Some loss of bone usually occurs naturally in both men and women after about age forty, but for some people, such as postmenopausal women, the decrease is more severe.

However, according to Dr. Louis V. Avioli, professor of medicine of Washington University School of Medicine, St. Louis, a recent study has revealed that 38 percent of men and 22 percent of women in their forties show little if any bone loss, so it is not inevitable.

Osteoporosis can occur in children and young adults, but most cases are seen after menopause in women. In fact, one out of every three or four women has the problem to some degree after menopause and should have help, according to one doctor interviewed. Women weighing less than 120 pounds develop osteoporosis at twice the rate of women weighing more than 140 pounds.

Osteoporosis can also be caused by calcium deficiency, either because there is not enough calcium in the diet or because the body does not absorb it properly. It can occur following prolonged treatment with corticosteroids. It can be made worse by immobilization, or insufficient physical activity, or several of these factors may occur together.

At first there are no symptoms that anything is going wrong; then the person begins to feel some back pain. Often before a diagnosis is even made, bone fractures can occur after what seems like the mildest bump or stress. Sometimes bones snap simply from carrying too much body weight. In fact, many times older people who have fallen and broken a hip have actually had a hip bone break spontaneously from a slight stress, *after which* they fall because of the broken hip. Sometimes vertebrae of the spine collapse or fracture, causing pain to radiate around the trunk, even to the buttocks or down the legs. Or strangely, the vertebrae can fracture and never even cause pain, so the person does not know anything has happened.

Persistent pain in the back is often due to osteoporosis. Usually there are periods of pain, followed by periods of improvement. If several vertebrae are collapsed, the person may become shorter. Or there may be the humping of the back and rounded shoulders so often seen in older people.

Diagnosis is usually aided by X-ray but can only be confirmed for sure by a biopsy sample taken from a bone. Unfortunately, by the time osteoporosis is seen on X-ray, a 35 to 50 percent bone loss may have already occurred.

TREATMENT

Doctors recommend a high intake of calcium supplements (in the form of tablets, dolomite, Os-Cal, or bone meal), in addition to a diet high in calcium (milk and cheese are good).

Supplements of vitamin D should be taken to ensure absorption of calcium by the intestines. (Check your doctor for the proper amount since vitamin D can accumulate in the body and result in toxic levels.)

Estrogen often is given. It does not rebuild deteriorated bone but may help prevent further bone loss in some but not all women. It can relieve pain and give an increased sense of well-being. If estrogen is taken, it should be taken cyclically, at as low a dose as possible for the shortest period of time, and only under a doctor's supervision.

As much physical activity as possible and an exercise program to stimulate bone growth and strengthen the back are recommended. Swimming and walking are especially good. If osteoporosis is severe, be careful of strenuous exercises that can break bones.

Medication for pain can be taken as needed.

Losing excess weight is often effective since it decreases the burden on the skeleton and leads to more physical activity.

Three drugs are sometimes used in the treatment of osteoporosis, although none of them has as yet been approved by the Food and Drug Administration for this indication: sodium fluoride, anabolic steroids, and calcitonin. Several doctors admitted using them with good results.

PREVENTION

Have an active life with plenty of regular exercise from an early age and throughout life. Do not ever let yourself become totally immobilized. Even if you have a chronic disease or ill health or are disabled, ask your doctor how you can exercise to a limited degree.

Eat a well-balanced diet, with plenty of calcium (at least 1 to 2 grams per day). Many doctors suggest that if calcium is not abundant in the diet, calcium supplements should be taken even at an early age. As one doctor said: "The more bone and stronger bone that is present at the age of thirty, the longer it would take before the bone loss leading to spinal vertebrae collapse and back pain occurs. In fact, if sufficient bone is accumulated during early years, the critical level may never be reached in a normal life span." Other doctors said that calcium supplements in early life are seldom necessary because calcium conservation in growing children is extremely efficient. Actually, says Dr. Avioli, it's not just the calcium, it's the calcium/phosphorus ratio in the diet that's important. If the phosphorus level is too high in relation to calcium, bone resorption tends to increase. The average American diet supplies about half as much calcium to phosphorus as is desirable. Carbonated soft drinks and animal protein contain much phosphorus, he said.

He recommends that everyone add calcium to the diet in the form of commercially available preparations such as Os-Cal (two to three tablets a day) to help retard bone loss.

28 What to Do for Shoulder Pain

Shoulder pain is a confusing pain, and in fact is often misdiagnosed as coming from the wrong cause. Sometimes the cause of the pain may be as simple as over-fatigue, chilling, or having held your head in an awkward position. The pain can be due to something actually occurring in the shoulder, such as an injury, bursitis, over-use of the muscles in painting or playing ball; or it can be referred pain that is felt in the shoulder but actually originates from a problem somewhere else, such as in the radiating pain from a heart attack or lung cancer or pain from the neck or back. Indeed, disorders in the neck present themselves much more frequently as shoulder pain than as neck pain.

Experts' tips on the best ways to tell when shoulder pain is referred from the neck. Referred pain is usually vague, nagging, felt in a broad, diffuse area. Referred pain from the neck may often be reproduced by moving the neck; locally caused pain will be reproduced by moving the shoulder. With referred pain, the shoulder joint has a full range of motion, but the neck may have some limitation of tilting or rotation. If you press your fingers deeply into the neck muscles and around the cervical spine, you may locate tender spots in the neck, indicating the pain originates there.

TREATMENT FOR SIMPLE SHOULDER PAIN

Rest the shoulder.
Apply cold compresses for the first day.

Take aspirin or other pain relievers.

Muscle relaxants are sometimes helpful.

On the second day and later, apply heat.

Warning: Be sure to avoid frozen shoulder. No matter what the cause of pain, even a hairline fracture, you should not let the shoulder become immobile. If you hold a shoulder in an inactive, stiff position for many days, it may become stiff for life. Move your arm and shoulder as much as you can each day, taking pain pills or applying heat to ease discomfort if necessary. Begin gently, increasing exercise each day until you can swing the arm freely in every direction.

If the pain is referred pain from a problem in the neck or elsewhere, treatment to the shoulder will have almost no effect. The cause of the pain, the original source, must be found and treated.

If the shoulder pain does not go away or lessen in two to three days, or if there is substantial swelling or suspicion of fracture or dislocation, see a physician for a thorough analysis.

EXERCISES TO RELIEVE TENSION IN THE SHOULDERS

Sitting or standing, grasp a bath towel at each end, pull it taut, and hold it in front of you at arm's length. Then raise the towel overhead, keeping elbows straight. Bend elbows and bring the towel down behind your back. Bring the towel back overhead and slowly forward again. Repeat 10 times. (You can do a variation of this with a broomstick, lifting the broomstick overhead, then bringing your arms behind your head. This is a good stretch exercise for bursitis.)

2. Stand with your feet slightly separated, bending forward, with your arms and head hanging loosely. Bring your arms around in a circle like a windmill, one arm at a time or both together, whichever is more comfortable for you. Repeat for about two minutes whenever neck, shoulders, or upper back become cramped. This loosens up stiff shoulder muscles.

3. Let your arms hang loosely at your sides. Rotate your shoulders in a circle by shrugging them as high as possible, then as far backward as possible, then relaxing. Hold head erect, not thrust forward. Repeat about 20 times to loosen shoulder and neck muscles.

AT-HOME SHOULDER TREATMENTS

1. This exercise is frequently recommended by osteopathic physicians after manipulation to help milk congestion out of muscles and help mobilize the shoulder. Sit in a chair with your head in a natural, relaxed position. A helper puts a hand firmly on your forehead, and you push your head against resistance as hard as possible in a forward direction, doing 10 pushes in a steady rhythm. Then push rhythmically in the same way against resistance in seven other directions: backward, to the left, to the right, then obliquely forward and right, forward and left, backward and right, backward and left. Do each 10 times. Then with the helper holding your head firmly between both hands, attempt to turn your head to the right against resistance, then to the left. Do 10 times each.

2. To strengthen your shoulder and loosen over-tight muscles, lie on your back on the floor with your knees bent, arms at your sides. Hold a weight in each hand (canned goods work well). Raise your arms up into the air, holding your elbows straight, and stretch your arms over your head to try to touch the floor, still keeping elbows straight. If you cannot touch all the way or keep your elbows straight, it indicates how tight your muscles are. Repeat 10 to 50 times once a day.

3. To strengthen an injured shoulder, stand erect and stretch both arms out to your sides in a T position with a rock, brick, or other weight in the hand of the injured arm. Swing your arm forward across your chest and return. Repeat 10 times. If this exercise causes pain, stop and use a lighter weight. Later, increase weight to that of a household iron.

29 What to Do for Neck Pain

Pain in the neck can be due to the flu, sitting in a draft, or having bad posture. It can be due to a pulled muscle, muscle strain or tension, arthritis, degeneration of a disk in a vertebra of the neck, or even cancer. Or it can be pain referred from nearby parts of the body.

EXPERTS' TIPS ON PREVENTING A STIFF, PAINFUL NECK

Avoid a forward thrust of the head and neck when walking or sitting.

Don't sit for a long time in a single position.

Don't sit under an air-conditioner or in any other draft.

Don't read or watch TV while lying down in bed or on a couch with your head at a sharp angle.

Try to correct your posture if it is faulty. Sit and stand relaxed but straight, and hold your neck straight, with the head centered over the shoulders.

Lower or raise work heights to keep all work at or near eye level. Use the stepladder for doing work above eye level.

Try to cut down tension.

Have your eyes and ears checked. If one side is stronger than the other side, it may cause you to constantly tilt your head to see or listen.

Make sure your car seat is adjusted properly so that you're not straining to see out the windshield.

Don't sleep face down with pressure on your neck.

Don't sleep while sitting up.

Choose a pillow that does not put stress on the neck or shoulders. Often it is best to maintain your head and neck in a neutral position so they are straight in line. But sometimes it feels better and does more good to keep your head just a little lower than your neck. Then there will be a gentle, natural traction effect on the neck muscles and joints because of the weight of the head. For some people, no pillow may be best, especially for those who sleep on their back.

Do back-strengthening exercises like the ones in this book. (The neck and the rest of the back are so closely related that weakness in one affects the other; in fact, a person who suffers problems in one area is likely to eventually suffer problems in the other.)

Check your bifocals. A person can stretch the neck awkwardly while reading or doing work at or above eye level. If you do a great deal of close work at eye level or higher, the problem can be solved by having the reading segment of your bifocals placed at the top of the lens instead of the bottom, or simply by using separate reading or work glasses.

How much do you talk on the telephone? Dr. Robert England, associate dean at Philadelphia College of Osteopathic Medicine, describes a case of a sixty-six-year-old man who had been in four hospitals under the care of neurologists for neck pain for nine months. "The man was near suicide because he could receive no relief," Dr. England said. After gentle stretching and other osteopathic manipulations over several weeks, he was almost pain-free. What caused the problem? "The only factor that might have caused the degenerative change as far as we could ascertain," says Dr. England, "was that the patient had held a telephone on his left shoulder for a minimum of eight hours almost daily for approximately twenty-five years."

EXERCISES TO RELIEVE NECK TENSION

1. Turn your head to look over the right shoulder as if watching an object go by at eye level. Then turn your head to look over the left shoulder. Keep your eyes on the same level. Turn your head as far as possible, but do not turn your shoulders or trunk. Repeat 5 times.

2. Cock your head to the right, moving your right ear down toward the right shoulder. Then move your left ear toward the left shoulder. Repeat 5 times as needed.

3. Put your neck through relaxed circles by putting your chin down toward your chest, then rotating your head in a complete circle around and back. Do 5 times in a clockwise direction, then 5 times in a counterclockwise direction. If you have pain each time your neck goes all the way back, change the exercise to half circles by putting your chin to your chest, then rotating your head to the right shoulder, then straight across to the left shoulder and then down to the chest again.

TREATMENTS FOR NECK PAIN

Take aspirin or other pain-killer.

Have a gentle soothing massage.

Rest in bed with the neck supported at a normal angle.

Avoid the vibration caused by automobile rides.

For sore muscles, apply superficial heat with heat lamp, heating pad, hot towel, sauna, whirlpool, long hot shower or bath. Deep heat from diathermy and ultrasound are sometimes used to reduce pain by increasing the blood supply to the area.

For bursitis or tendinitis, use cold or ice packs to help shrink inflammation and reduce pain.

For more severe pain, a cervical collar, muscle relaxants or sedatives may be helpful. (Try not to use a collar for more than 10–14 days because muscles and joints may get stiff.)

Pain can often be relieved by having a physician apply firm pressure over a muscle or ligament trigger point, injecting procaine or hydrocortisone into the area, or using a vapor-coolant spray like fluorimethane. Acupuncture can be helpful also.

Some doctors recommend traction; some feel it does more harm than good. One doctor cautioned that after an injury stretching and traction should not be done before one week to allow healing of tissues.

Gentle osteopathic manipulation carefully performed may often help neck pain unsuccessfully treated by other means.

After the acute stage has passed, it is recommended that exercises should be performed to strengthen neck muscles.

See a doctor immediately if neck pain travels down the arm, an arm is numb or tingly, if there is high fever, or if pain is severe, persists or recurs frequently.

A NEW OSTEOPATHIC MANIPULATION FOR THE NECK

Dr. Milton Mintz, of Denville, New Jersey, uses this technique for wryneck and stiff, sore neck. The patient sits in a chair with the head turned to the left. The practitioner, standing behind, places his right hand on the patient's chin and the left hand on the back of the neck, and rotates upward and backward, extending and stretching the neck by pulling. Usually you hear a popping sound as the ligaments stretch, says Dr. Mintz, and by the time the patient leaves the office he is pain-free. Mintz strongly warns that you don't try this on your own. It could cause injury. It should only be done by a physician skilled in manipulation.

IF YOU HAVE CERVICAL DISK DISEASE

You can have a disk problem in the neck just as you can in the lower back. For years it may appear as a stiff neck; then the pain increases and may radiate from the neck to the shoulder, down the arm, and even to the fingers.

About 80 percent of all patients can be managed by conservative therapy: bed rest, aspirin, and muscle relaxants.

Sometimes traction is helpful.

In some cases, surgery is necessary to relieve pressure on the nerve roots.

One surgeon said he found no benefit from a soft cervical collar, and usually hard cervical collars did not fit well. He recommended one- or two-piece styrofoam collars carefully fitted if the neck needs supporting.

Note: Most people over age sixty have some bone changes in the neck that can be seen on X-ray. These are areas of wear or roughening of the surface of the cartilage and bone, which may not necessarily lead to uncomfortable symptoms.

A NEW CERVICAL COLLAR

Dr. J. DeWitt Fox, director of the Neurologic Center of Los Angeles, has designed a cervical collar with contoured support to reduce neck tension and pain. In colors. Available from Fox Instruments, 7080 Hollywood Boulevard, Los Angeles, California 90028. $37.50.

A DO-IT-YOURSELF CHIROPRACTOR'S HEAD-LIFT FOR THE NECK

Place your hands on the sides of your neck and use both hands as though trying to lift the head off the shoulders. Lift straight up and a little forward, never backward. Turn your head to the left, then the right, and try to lift even harder. Continue as many movements as are comfortable. The head-lift is designed to release nerve pressures in the neck.

AN INEXPENSIVE NECK SUPPORT

To relieve pain, you can make a collar support with a hand towel. Fold the towel lengthwise four times and wrap it snugly around the person's neck. It should encircle the neck about one and one-half times, overlapping beneath the chin. Fasten with two large safety pins.

Or you can make a neck support from newspaper folded to approximately the height of the neck and covered with a nylon stocking or bandage material, or from a stocking filled with polyurethane foam.

Any cervical collar, whether purchased or made at home, should be placed in such a way that the head is held comfortably in a position that does not over-extend the neck and force the chin upward.

EXERCISES TO STRENGTHEN THE NECK

When neck symptoms become severe, surgery is sometimes performed to fuse the neck vertebrae in order to eliminate symptoms. But four out of five of these operations can be avoided with a proper exercise program, says Dr. Jay A. Wiersma, osteopathic physician of Grand Rapids, Michigan.

After an acute attack of neck pain he recommends the following exercises be done, as soon as the person can tolerate mild activity.

The exercises were developed by Dr. Alfred B. Swanson, of

Blodgett Memorial Hospital in Grand Rapids, and have been used by Dr. Wiersma with excellent success for the past ten years. The exercises are performed with a bath towel after a hot shower or bath.

1. Tense the muscles in front of the neck, pull the chin down, shake the head in a "no-no" rotation on the chest.

2. Place a folded towel behind the neck, strongly pull the towel up and forward with the chin down, rotate the head slightly.

3. Place a towel across the forehead. Tense the muscles in front of the neck with resistance from the towel, rotate the head with the chin on the chest.

Dr. Mark D. Brown, back surgeon at the University of Miami School of Medicine, and head of the new back clinic there, uses strengthening exercises both before patients undergo neck surgery and to rehabilitate muscles after surgery. He recommends the following neck exercises.

1. Grasp both hands behind the head, keeping the neck in a neutral aligned position. Pull forward with the arms and push back with the head to the count of 3. Relax. Repeat 10 times.

2. Then put the hand against the side of the head and push the head against the hand for resistance. Do on both sides.

3. Finally place the palm of the hand on the forehead. Press back with the arm and forward with the head.

You should do all three exercises only within the limits of pain, Dr. Brown cautions.

THE SCALENUS ANTICUS SYNDROME

Many times persons with this syndrome of persistent pain extending from the neck into the arms and fingers are thought to be neurotic because of the puzzling nature of their symptoms. The pain is often described as dull and aching, but may also be sharp and burning. It is often made worse by turning the head. It may not occur with some activities, but then is brought on by others—those it turns out that cause the arms to be elevated for prolonged periods, such as painting ceilings and high walls.

The scalenus anticus is a muscle stretched between the neck and the first rib. The arteries and nerves to the arm are right next to the scalenus anticus muscle and their interaction with the muscle seems to cause the pain.

Schoolteachers who write on blackboards, auto mechanics working over their heads, trap shooters, and many others suffer the syndrome because they must hold their arms high for long periods during their work or activity.

If the problem is not treated, the arms may become weak or numb. Doctors usually recommend the correction of poor posture, weight reduction if the person is fat, proper support for oversize breasts, and neck exercises. Sometimes an anesthetic can be injected into the neck muscle. Sometimes surgery to cut the muscle is necessary to release the pressure.

30 What You Should Know about Whiplash Injury

Most whiplash injuries come from car accidents when a person is suddenly snapped in one direction, then the opposite. But there are other causes too. A person misses a step in the dark, suddenly falls forward, then recoils. A swimmer is caught by a breaker and is bent backward, then forward, by the impact of a wave. A youngster on a trampoline loses his balance and throws his body. An amusement park ride throws you one way, then another.

A 3,500-pound car traveling at only ten miles per hour can transmit a blow amounting to twenty-five tons when it hits the rear of another car. A head weighing only eight or nine pounds, mounted on a flexible neck, is quite vulnerable to sudden changes of force of direction. The head snaps forward or backward or to the side with several tons of force.

WHIPLASH SYMPTOMS

At first you may have none at all. After a few hours you may have a little soreness, stiffness, nausea. The next day there may be headache and more stiffness.

Usually after two days or so, the shock produced from snapping the body back and forth begins to result in major symptoms: pounding headache, nausea, dizziness, and pain in the shoulders, arms, hands, chest, back, even the pelvis. There also may be blurred vision, aching eyeballs, or disturbances in hearing. After a

225

week or so, the patient often manifests depression, anxiety, or anger.

DIAGNOSIS

Because the injury is mostly to the ligaments, muscles, tendons, and joint capsules, *the whiplash injury will not show up on X-ray film.* The doctor will still do an X-ray to check for fractures or dislocations, but the extent of the injury is largely determined by the doctor feeling the muscles with his fingers, checking for muscle spasm, reflexes, whether you have any loss of sensation, and checking how much range of motion you have, and what movements cause you pain.

HOW TO TELL WHEN SOMEONE'S FAKING

In *Medical Trial Techniques Quarterly,* Dr. R. Bingham outlines the following points to watch for in a faker.

1. He resists the examiner.

2. He tolerates very little discomfort, jerks away when touched, and says it hurts.

3. He complains of many areas of pain.

4. His headaches are "terrible," but he does not mention that they are associated with eye strain, or hearing or visual disturbances, which usually are present in severe whiplash.

5. When a pinwheel is run over the skin for diagnosis, he says it hurts terribly.

6. When you ask him to squeeze a dynamometer to measure grip, he grips only with his fingers, has a wide variation in grip strength, and reaches only a third the power of a normal person.

7. He doesn't know, and so doesn't show, the most typical signs—that the motions of extension and rotation are the most painful and the most limited.

(Long-lasting symptoms do not necessarily mean a person is faking. Symptoms frequently last for months, sometimes years. In one study, 85 percent of those followed up after two years still had some symptoms.)

TREATMENT

During the first twenty-four hours. Cold packs or ice massage for seven minutes every hour; aspirin or other painkillers, nausea medication if nausea is present; rest and elimination of movement to prevent further stretching of nerves and tissue.

After the first twenty-four hours. Hot wet packs or hot showers; a cervical collar to give support and ease pressure on nerve roots; manipulation by a physician trained in osteopathic techniques. Sometimes medication is given to relax muscle spasm, or injections are given at trigger points to relieve pain. In some cases spinal traction is recommended, especially in the first seventy-two hours. Hydrotherapy or diathermy may be given.

Acupuncture has been reported to be useful. Ultrasound can act as a micromassage, increases circulation, and reduces calcium deposits, scar tissue, and bruising.

Rest is essential, since injured nerves and tissue can be stretched painfully with ordinary movement. The sufferer should especially limit activities involving the head and arms, should always bend the knees in picking up anything from the floor, and should not reach above the head. If symptoms are persistent, the patient may need complete bed rest for a week to remove the weight of the head from the neck. Some are helped by resting the head on a pillow a little higher than the neck to relieve pressure.

Vitamin therapy is used by some physicians to counteract stress, and usually includes vitamin B_1 and B_{12} plus vitamin C with bioflavinoid and rutin.

Avoid riding in cars, since this aggravates neck pain.

BEST WAYS TO PREVENT WHIPLASH

Don't tailgate (90 percent of whiplash injuries are the result of rearend collisions).

Don't let anyone tailgate you; stay to the right and let them pass; or if you want to take a leisurely drive, take a more scenic side road instead of a busy highway.

Watch for sudden changes in traffic conditions ahead and be prepared for quick stops.

Allow plenty of room for stops at high speed. It takes longer than you think.

Make sure your brakes are in good condition.

Use proper signals to indicate turns or stops. Keep your eye on the rear-view mirror to see that the car behind you is reacting to your signals.

If you think you are about to be hit from the back, move ahead whatever distance you can, or move quickly off to the side shoulder of the road. Protect your head and neck with your arms; fall across the seat for extra protection.

Use safety belts, and have a properly adjusted headrest.

Don't drive more than fifty-five to sixty miles per hour.

31 Other Special Back Problems and What to Do for Them

OSTEOMALACIA

Osteomalacia means softening of the bone. It is primarily due to deficiency of vitamin D and calcium, or an upset in their absorption and metabolism in the body. It is similar to rickets, can occur in children or adults, is especially well known in the groups of women in the Orient who during pregnancy are kept indoors, seldom seeing the sun, and who subsist on diets low in calcium. The disease is not as common in the United States as in Britain, but anyone who does not get much sunlight or take vitamin D risks developing osteomalacia. "It's far more common than realized," says Dr. Gregory Mundy, of the University of Connecticut. In fact, he estimates that 20 percent of older persons in the United States with osteoporosis also have osteomalacia.

People may have the condition because of improper diet, poor absorption of nutrients, or operations that have removed part of the stomach. Persons with kidney, pancreas, or liver disorders are also likely to get osteomalacia, as are alcoholics and persons who take anticonvulsant drugs over long periods. Two chemicals—fluorides and diphosphonates—can also induce osteomalacia.

The softening of the bone goes on all over the body, but occurs particularly in the spine, ribs, shoulder, pelvis, and legs. Bone pain in those areas may range from a dull ache to severe pain, generally beginning with tenderness and pain in the lower back. The bone tenderness is felt with pressure. There may also

229

be muscle weakness. Later there may be humping of the back and shortening of the spine, or side-curving of the spine. The patient may have difficulty in climbing stairs or getting out of a chair, or may have a waddling gait.

The disease is often mistaken for osteoporosis or arthritis.

Treatment

Vitamin D taken daily by mouth or weekly by injection.

A good diet which includes milk, eggs, butter, or margarine.

Calcium supplements.

Pain and weakness usually disappear within four to eight weeks after starting treatment. Usually high doses are used at first, then are reduced to a maintenance dose as healing begins. Both vitamin D and calcium should be taken under the direction of a physician since too much vitamin D can be dangerous, and calcium needs to be balanced properly with other minerals. In some cases, phosphorus is also needed, doctors told us.

Any major deformities may have to be corrected by traction or surgery, or both.

Prevention

Get plenty of sunshine for vitamin D.

Eat plenty of dairy foods, or take fish liver oil regularly.

Have adequate amounts of calcium in the diet, or take calcium supplements.

Elderly persons, patients taking long-term anticonvulsants, persons who have stomach surgery, and those who do not spend much time outdoors should particularly ensure a proper diet, take calcium supplements, and get plenty of sunshine.

Note: There is also a rare form of osteomalacia caused by a tumor. The treatment for this is the surgical removal of the tumor. According to doctors at Duke University, an experimental drug that is a form of vitamin D can prevent painful symptoms if the tumor should grow back again.

PAGET'S DISEASE

In this disease of the bone, also called osteitis deformans, bones increase in size and sometimes shape, and have a slightly different internal structure and architecture. It is a chronic disease which begins very slowly, often starting in middle age but not becoming apparent until age sixty or later. In many instances the changes are very mild, and progress remains almost stationary for years. In fact, in most patients there are no symptoms and the diagnosis is determined when signs of the bone changes show up unexpectedly on X-ray studies taken for other reasons. About two million men and women in the United States have the disorder.

The disorder is not life-threatening, but because of the irregular structure of the affected bone, the bone is often weak, so that there may be easy fracturing or crippling. One bone may be affected, or the entire skeleton. Most commonly affected are the back, pelvis, skull, and leg bones. Pain in the bones of the back, hips, or legs may be difficult to distinguish from the pain of osteoarthritis, which, in fact, is often associated with Paget's disease. The spine is almost always involved, and often seems to shrink and become shorter, with increased curving in the front and back. The skull also seems thicker and there is frequent bowing of the legs.

Occasionally, in advanced cases, there may be compression of the nerves in the spine, causing paralysis because of nerve damage, but this complication is very rare.

Treatment. Until recently there was no effective treatment, but now there are several effective agents for relieving symptoms. However, they are still classified by the FDA as investigational drugs. Most patients need no treatment at all.

REITER'S SYNDROME

The cause of Reiter's syndrome is unknown, but there is some suspicion that it is caused by a bacterium since it often follows an intestinal or genitourinary infection. At other times there seems to be no connection to an infection at all.

Symptoms include a strange three-way combination: inflammation of the urethra, inflammation of the membrane of the eye or other mucous membranes, and arthritis, including arthritis of the spine. It can occur at any age, even in children, but is most common between the ages of twenty and forty. There seems to be a hereditary tendency to develop the disease. The key to diagnosis is the three-way symptoms of the urinary system, the eyes, and the joints at the same or nearly the same time, usually within a few days or weeks of each other. Joint pain may occur in the extremities, especially the feet, or may appear as low back pain. Arthritis pain usually lasts about three months, but may last longer. There may be repeated episodes, which may or may not be preceded by sexual exposure.

Treatment. Aspirin and other anti-inflammatory drugs such as indomethacin and Butazolidin. In *severe* cases, immunosuppressive agents such as azathioprine and methotrexate help relieve symptoms, but these should only be used in extremely serious cases that have not responded to other treatment since there are many side effects to these drugs.

RICKETS

Rickets is a disease in which there is faulty laying down of minerals in cartilage. The growing bone does not become properly calcified. By definition, it cannot occur after the bones have formed and fused, and so occurs only in children, never in adults. Rickets can develop because of poor diet, because a child does not get the sunshine necessary for the absorption of vitamin D, or because of some upset in metabolism or digestion which interferes with absorption and utilization of vitamin D in the body. The abnormalities can occur in all bones, including the spine.

Infants with rickets are restless and sleep poorly, often have a bald spot on the head from moving it constantly in their restlessness. Diagnosis is made by X-ray, which can show the changes in the bones.

Treatment. Large doses of vitamin D supplements taken daily, with first signs of improvement occurring in about ten days. After about one month, doses can be reduced to maintenance levels.

32 Special Back and Neck Problems of Children and What Can Be Done to Help Them

CONGENITAL WRYNECK (Torticollis)

In this birth disorder, the neck is twisted and the head is cocked to the side. Some physicians believe it is due to difficulty during labor and delivery. Others believe it is due to muscle imbalance in the developing fetus. Whatever the cause, one of the neck muscles is contracted so the head is held to one side.

Diagnostic clues. Several days after birth a lump is sometimes noticeable in the muscle area on the side of the neck. At age three or four, tilting of the head may become noticeable. The ear on the lower side seems to be shorter and wider and appears to stand out from the head. For some unknown reason, the abnormality is on the right side in three out of four children who have the problem, and 20 percent of the victims also have congenital hip problems.

It is essential to detect the neck abnormality early so exercises can be started in infancy or early childhood to prevent the development of severe wryneck symptoms and the possible facial deformities that can otherwise occur. (The child often sleeps with the affected side down, so the face is flattened on one side where it usually presses against the bed.)

Only a physician can diagnose this ailment, and at no time should parents attempt to treat the condition without direct medical supervision. About 90 percent of children respond to stretching exercises alone. Occasionally surgery is necessary to remove part of the neck muscle.

233

An easy aid: Position crib toys so the infant has to stretch his neck in reaching for the toy. Be sure the child does not always sleep on one side.

JUVENILE RHEUMATOID ARTHRITIS

See page 183.

OSTEOGENESIS IMPERFECTA

In this rather rare metabolic disorder the bones are very fragile and will often break at the slightest impact. There is no cure but there is evidence that large amounts of vitamin C and magnesium can help patients somewhat.

Dr. Clive C. Solomons, of the University of Colorado Medical Center, reported that daily doses of magnesium oxide significantly helped more than half of the children whom he treated.

Then three years later, in 1974, Dr. Diann Kurz and Dr. Edward J. Eyring reported in *Pediatrics* that high doses of vitamin C (1,000 to 2,000 milligrams per day) also helped. Patients, from newborns to a fifteen-year-old, were followed for ten to forty-three months. *All* of them, the doctors said, had a reduced number of fractures and were able to increase physical activity and have a normal life. The authors point out that this was not a controlled experiment; the children were not matched to others with the disease who did not receive vitamin C, and the number of patients was small. However, they feel the results are promising and warrant further investigation.

Both vitamin C and magnesium affect zinc levels and an enzyme in the body which influences bones and growth and may be the clue to the mechanism if future research proves that vitamin C and magnesium actually work to help children with this disease.

ROUNDBACK (Also called kyphosis or Scheuermann's disease)

Many people have children with this condition and don't realize it, thinking their child only has poor posture. But the condition is actually caused by wedge-shaped vertebrae that cause the spine to curve forward. Untreated, the problem can produce unsightly deformity and lifelong back problems. Early recognition and proper treatment can produce superior results.

If a child is seriously stoop-shouldered, a physician should be consulted.

If the condition is not treated during adolescence, it can definitely be expected to progress.

Treatment usually involves a compound approach: exercises to loosen contracted muscles, sometimes bed rest and traction to loosen muscles, then application of a plaster cast or a Milwaukee brace to correct the curvature. The exercise program includes exercises to reduce excess curving of the back, as our program does, and to correct the round-shouldered slumping by hyperextension of the trunk. In fact, three exercises in our program are specifically used by many orthopedic specialists to correct this condition: the Pelvic Tilt, the Straight Leg Raise, and the Chest Raise.

If exercise alone is used for treatment, frequent X-rays should be taken to make sure the curvature is being brought under control. Any sign of progression of the condition means treatment with a Milwaukee brace should begin immediately.

Surgery rarely is needed.

SCOLIOSIS (Curvature of the spine)

This deformity was recognized as far back as the time of Hippocrates, who first applied the term "scoliosis" (Greek for crooked). *Recent school screenings indicate that 10 to 12 percent of youngsters screened have the deformity in one form or another.*

The sideways curve of the spine may appear gradually at first, then progresses rapidly in a very short time, becoming worse and worse with the growth of the spine. Usually there isn't any pain (although there may be a dull ache); the spine simply becomes more and more curved as the child grows older. At first it is barely noticeable—one hip may appear a little higher than the other, and the ribs and shoulder blades may start to curve out of line. But if the deformity is not corrected before age seventeen or eighteen, when spinal growth stops, it will remain for the rest of a person's life. It can crowd vital organs, produce a hunched back, and even cause death.

Scoliosis can be caused by polio, muscular dystrophy, rheumatoid arthritis, cerebral palsy, and spinal injuries. It may also be a delayed consequence of congenital hip dislocation, so the parents of a child born with this disorder should be particularly alert later on for the appearance of spinal curvature. But in 90 percent of the cases, the cause is unknown.

Note: Many children with scoliosis also have abnormalities of the genitourinary system. Many doctors recommend that any child with scoliosis should automatically have routine intravenous X-ray studies of the genitourinary system.

For most scoliosis victims, some form of corrective brace—usually one called a Milwaukee brace—is prescribed. The brace consists of a girdle that fits around the hips and three vertical bars that attach at the top to a neck ring and throat mold. Early models were made of leather and steel; now models are lightweight aluminum and plastic. The brace helps the spine grow straight.

One doctor gave these guidelines: All curves of more than 15 to 30 degrees should be treated, as should any curving that becomes progressively worse with time. The brace should be able to maintain curvature under 50 degrees. Curves above 60 degrees should be corrected with surgery that fuses the vertebrae together. "Progression must *never* be allowed," we were told.

Casts instead of braces are often used in infants.

If a brace causes sore spots, the adjustment should be made by a physician. Never make changes yourself.

Once started, a brace is usually worn at all times, or for twenty-three out of every twenty-four hours. Patients can often be allowed to participate in sports. Swimming is greatly encouraged, and many doctors say swimming for at least an hour a day will help correct the problem. The brace should be worn for at least a year; then the wearing time is gradually reduced by about three hours every three months. The brace should not be stopped completely as long as the child continues to grow. Curvature tends to worsen during the rapid growth of adolescence, so children should be watched especially during this time. If a teen-ager refuses to wear the brace, fusion is almost always necessary.

The most common operation for scoliosis was developed in the 1960s by Dr. Paul Harrington, of Houston, and is now performed on most patients requiring surgery. Doctors implant thin steel rods next to the spine under the back muscles and attach the rods to the vertebrae with metal hooks that are then tightened—much like braces for the teeth—to force the spine to straighten. At the same time the spine is fused to give it additional strength. Patients who undergo surgery may spend up to four weeks in the hospital and up to ten months in a body cast at home afterward, but the results are excellent. Patients can lead completely normal lives. Youngsters can participate in sports. Women can have normal pregnancies a year or two after surgery.

A new experimental treatment, electrospinal stimulation for mild scoliosis among young children, produces improvement at home while the child sleeps. Electrodes are buried in the spinal muscles on the convex side of the curve and are attached to an implanted "spinal pacemaker" which stimulates the muscles at intervals during the night during sleep. A clinical trial of the method shows encouraging results. It is available at ten or twelve medical centers in the United States for experimental use.

A Simple Test for Scoliosis

Have the child strip to the waist. Carefully observe the child's back while he or she stands erect, feet together, arms hanging straight down.

Are the shoulder levels unequal?

Are the two sides of the hip unequal?

Is the waistline uneven?

Is the spine curved to one side or the other?

Is one shoulder blade more prominent than the other?

Is the distance between the arms and body unequal?

Next, have the child turn around and face you, then bend forward at a right angle, with legs straight, feet together, and arms hanging straight down from the shoulder.

Is there a difference in level between the two sides of the back?

Is there a hump on one side of the upper back and another hump on the other side of the lower back?

If you answer "yes" to any of these questions, there is a possibility of scoliosis, and you should have your child examined as soon as possible by your family doctor, pediatrician, or orthopedic surgeon.

Never attempt to correct a curvature of the spine yourself. This condition must be treated by a physician as soon as its presence is suspected.

Moiré Shadows—A New Technique for Detecting Scoliosis

A simple, innovative way of finding hidden cases of scoliosis is a screening technique that truly uses a screen—a screen of threads that casts contour-like shadows on a child's back. Called moiré photography, the technique shows whether the contours of the back are normal and symmetrical or are abnormally out of line.

Because it is cheap, quick, easy to do, and reliable, it is a natural for school screening programs, says one of the developers of the test, Dr. Gordon W. D. Armstrong, orthopedic surgeon at the University of Ottawa, Canada. The moiré technique shows a pattern of curved lines that outline body deformities, he says. Any difference in structure is easily seen by the different shape and size of the curve patterns on different sides of the spine.

The technique is twice as accurate as examining a child when he or she is bending over, he says. It picked up 94 percent of cases of scoliosis in a pilot program with schoolchildren in Ottawa (later confirmed by X-ray), he reports.

Dr. R. Kirklin Ashley, president of the Scoliosis Research Society, calls the technique promising but says it is still in the investigational stage.

Special Exercise Program for Scoliosis

The following exercise program has been described by Dr. Arthur A. Michele, professor and chairman of the department of orthopedic surgery at New York Medical College, in his book *Orthotherapy* (M. Evans, New York, 1971). Dr. Michele reports that he has had great success with these exercises but cautions that no exercise program for scoliosis should be done without permission and supervision from your doctor.

Spinal rotator muscle stretch and strengthening exercise. Kneel on the floor. Put your right knee as far forward as you can and stretch your left leg straight out behind you. Brace yourself with your left arm, and lift your right arm out to the side so that it is on a line with your shoulder. Bend the right arm at the elbow so it forms a right angle and your fingers are pointing over your head. From this position pull your bent right arm strongly back and turn your head and trunk to the right. The pull on your right arm and shoulder should be strong enough to turn the head and trunk with it. Relax into a starting position. Repeat pull smartly to the count of 4. Rest briefly. Repeat cycle 5 to 10 times, then switch leg and arm positions and repeat 5 to 10 times with left arm.

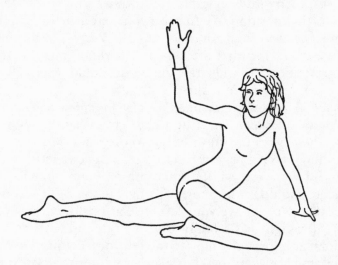

Stretching and strengthening exercise for the spinal column and shoulder musculature. Starting position—on your knees, thighs perpendicular to the floor, head and chest resting very near the floor, arms straight out over your head. Keeping your face and chest down, arms stretched out, shuffle your knees forward one at a time in tiny two- to three-inch "steps." Inching forward in this way, move your whole body in a circle on the floor to the right, then in a circle to the left. This may take as much as five minutes per circle.

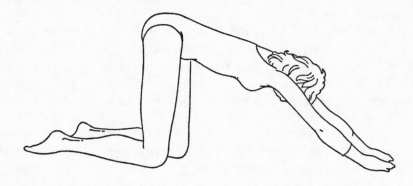

Strengthening exercise for spine, shoulder, shoulder blade, and hip musculature. Get down on the floor on your hands and knees. Simultaneously raise your right arm straight forward and raise your left leg straight backward. Hold for a count of 4 then return to the starting position. Then raise your left arm and right leg in the same way and hold for a count of 4. You will find that your body is inching forward after each lift when you return to the starting position. In this fashion you should gradually move across the floor for about three minutes.

Stretching and strengthening exercise for spine, shoulder blade, and hip musculature. Kneel and clasp your hands behind your head so the elbows fan straight out to the sides. Move your right knee as far forward as you can and stretch your left leg straight out behind you. You will be squatting on your right foot. Turn your head, shoulders, and torso strongly to the right and hold for a count of 4. Now, move your left knee as far forward as you can, stretch your right leg straight out behind, and turn your head, shoulders, and torso strongly to the left for a count of 4. You will find that you are again making a series of "steps" across the floor. Alternating sides, continue moving across the floor in this fashion for one to three minutes.

Spinal column stretch and abdominal strengthening. Sit on the floor and spread your legs as far apart as you can. Keep your knees straight. Bend forward at the waist and stretch your arms straight out over your head between your legs. Bounce forward in this fashion 10 times. Now tuck your right arm behind your back and stretch your left hand out toward your right foot. Bounce toward your right foot 10 times. Change sides. Tuck your left arm behind your back and reach your right hand for your left foot and bounce 10 times.

Stretching exercise for hamstrings, low back and spinal musculature. Stand with your feet widely separated, legs straight. Bend forward from the waist and reach for your right foot with your left hand, while swinging your right arm straight back and up. Bounce, reaching for your right foot with your left hand each time, to the count of 4. Return to the starting position. Bend forward from your waist and reach for your left foot with your right hand, swinging your left arm behind you. Bounce to the count of 4. Repeat this cycle 5 times.

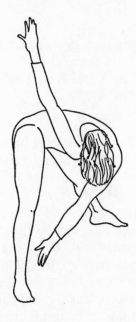

Strengthening exercise for low back and hip musculature. Kneel so your thighs are perpendicular to the floor. Rest your face on folded hands on the floor. Lift your left leg straight up as high off the floor as you can. Aim to get the lifted leg on a straight line with your trunk. Return to the starting position. Repeat the left leg lift 10 times. Return to the starting position and lift your right leg 10 times.

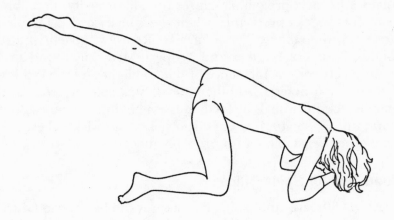

For Further Help

Local chapter meetings, a newsletter, and help in setting up school screening programs are available from the Scoliosis Association, 1 Penn Plaza, New York, New York 10001.

SPINA BIFIDA

This congenital defect is obvious at birth; the infant sometimes has an opening in the spine or a projection of the spinal cord to the outside. This is serious because it exposes a part of the nervous system to the outside. Modern medical treatment can help many victims to lead nearly normal lives.

Some of the children also have a hunchback condition. This often can be helped in early years by braces, and in later years by a new technique just developed by Dr. Douglas W. McKay, chief of orthopedics at Children's Hospital National Medical Center in Washington. He has successfully treated the hunchback condition of nine spinal bifida children by implanting a steel plate into the back and attaching the backbone to it to keep the back straight. The operation is best done at ages 6 to 10, he says.

If a child is born with spina bifida or with anencephaly (part of the brain missing at birth), the parents have 1 chance in 20 that any future children will be born with spina bifida. If such a defect occurs in two children in a family, the risk for a future defect is doubled.

An unproven theory recently proposed is that eating blighted potatoes in early pregnancy causes the abnormality, probably at about four weeks pregnancy when the spinal cord is first being formed in the embryo. Dr. James H. Renwick, geneticist at the London School of Hygiene and Tropical Medicine, found a relationship between the incidence of potato blight and the incidence of these birth defects. Another doctor was able to produce the same defects in animals by feeding them blighted potatoes. Blight shows up on potatoes as dark spots. Dr. Renwick believes that some other vegetable is also probably involved.

Blood Test for Spina Bifida

About 80 percent of spina bifida cases can be detected during pregnancy at sixteen to eighteen weeks. Called alpha-feto-protein

(AFP), the test can identify women at risk of carrying an infant with the congenital defect. If the diagnosis is confirmed by further tests, the mother can elect to have an abortion.

The test of the mother's blood is also 90 percent effective in detecting cases of fetuses who will be born without brains.

SPONDYLOLISTHESIS

This condition occurs when one vertebra slides forward and overhangs the vertebra below it. Sometimes it occurs in children aged three or four, but more frequently it is seen during the rapid growth period between five and eight. The cause of the slow slippage is unknown. Some doctors believe it is caused by muscle imbalance; others believe it is a birth defect, a congenital weakness of one of the vertebrae that is made to slip by body weight. It may also be brought on by injury. The vertebra may slide only slightly out of position, or it may be totally displaced.

The back muscles often tense up to withstand the strain and may become very rigid. The child may or may not have pain; if there is pain, it is generally in the lower back area, or it may be in the buttocks and thighs. Symptoms are aggravated by strenuous activity and are relieved by rest. The child also often has tightness of the hamstring muscles in the legs, with a typical posture of bending slightly forward with flexed hips and knees.

Diagnostic clues. The child may have difficulty raising a leg without bending the knee, may not be able to flex the hips with the knees extended, and may have to squat and bend at the knees to pick something up. And there may be a strange way of walking—a stiff-legged and mincing gait one doctor calls a "pelvic waddle."

Treatment. Usually a surgical corset or brace to support the weakened and strained spinal area will give the displaced vertebra a chance to stabilize. For an acute attack—bed rest and aspirin. A medically supervised program of exercise therapy to strengthen the muscles of the back and pelvis, such as the one in this book, can help prevent further damage. If exercise is not successful, surgery may be necessary.

SPONDYLOLYSIS

In this condition, which can lead to spondylolisthesis, there is actual breakdown of one of the vertebrae. There may be a heredity factor, since in some families one fourth to two thirds of the family members are so afflicted, especially in some Eskimo tribes. It can also be caused by a fracture of part of the vertebrae following injury, or even from stress, such as in soldiers carrying heavy backpacks or persons performing exercises they are not accustomed to.

Because of the fracture and breakdown, some people also get a slippage of the vertebra like that which occurs in spondylolithesis.

In children the problem usually occurs from about age seven or eight to age twenty. About 5 percent of the general population have the condition, but most never develop symptoms of any kind.

Most doctors interviewed felt that children without symptoms could engage in whatever activities they wished, and did not need to be restricted in any way.

For those with mild backaches or tightness of the hamstring muscles in the leg, vigorous activities that could cause injury should be restricted, and the child should do back-strengthening exercises as outlined in the exercise program in this book.

Those few patients with more severe complaints may require bed rest, traction, or medication for pain. In a very small percentage of patients who do not respond to exercise, surgery may be required to stabilize the spine.

Doctors interviewed also recommended that children and adolescents with the condition have annual X-rays to keep a check on the condition.

33 When Surgery Is Necessary

DO YOU NEED THE OPERATION?

Surgeons in Long Beach, California, are using psychological tests to determine who will or will not be most likely to get relief from back pain with surgery. Psychologist Patrick Rocchio and surgeon Leon Wiltse tested 130 patients over three years and found that psychological tests were able to prevent some useless operations. They used a standard test called the Minnesota Multiphasic Personality Inventory and found that if patients scored 85 or more in the hypochondriasis and hysteria sections, they had only a 10 percent chance of getting good relief from an operation. If the patients had a standard score of 54 or less, there was a 90 percent chance of success.

When back surgery is of greatest benefit. According to the doctors interviewed, surgery is most successful when the patient has a large ruptured disk and enormous pain. But surgery is not inevitable, they stressed. About 80 percent of patients with a slipped disk do well with exercise and other conservative treatment and never need surgery. The other 20 percent have surgery because they want faster relief or because their particular disability requires it.

ANSWERS TO QUESTIONS MOST OFTEN ASKED ABOUT BACK SURGERY

When should surgery be done? It should be done as a last resort only after a thorough exercise program has been tried. Because any kind of surgery carries some risk, surgery should never be done unless necessary.

What is the most common kind of back surgery? Removal of a disk.

Why do you remove a disk? If it is bulging and pressing on a nerve, causing excruciating pain. Removing the disk removes the pressure and the cause of the pain.

What happens to the hole? In the space where the disk was, the body forms scar tissue and the space is filled in. There is no way to replace the disk.

How many disk operations are done? Some 110,000 spinal disk operations are performed each year in the United States by neurosurgeons, and many more by orthopedic surgeons. In Europe, the percentage of operations for back pain is much lower. Many doctors feel that too many such operations are performed in the United States.

What happens if the disk operation fails? The patients who get to physicians who give them corrective exercises often still do well. Others may end up in special pain clinics or having cordotomies (cutting the spinal cord) to treat the failure of disk surgery. Besides other complications, almost 100 percent of male patients who have cordotomies are left with total or near-total sexual impotence.

What is spinal fusion? This is an alternate surgical technique sometimes used when there is degeneration of a disk in the spine, but usually for other spinal weaknesses. In fusion, two or three joints are fused together by bridging and stiffening the vertebrae with a bone graft that actually makes one bone out of two. Bone chips are usually taken from another part of the body (usually the hip bone) and grafted or joined together with the affected vertebrae to form a solid, nonflexible section of the spine. The rest of the back remains flexible and you are able to bend and move normally. Many fusions, but not all, involve the insertion of a slender, stainless-steel rod, called a Harrington rod, along the affected area of the spine. It attaches to the top and bottom vertebrae to help hold the spine rigid while the bone graft heals. This operation is not used as much as it once was for disk degeneration, since comparative studies show it just does not do that much good. Most doctors believe that fusing one level doesn't protect other levels of the spine. The technique is still very useful when there is weakness of a single vertebra or two, or where there is a slipping of the vertebrae.

What is arthrodesis? This is the scientific name for fusion of two joint surfaces.

How long does it take to recover from a spinal fusion operation? A typical operation means about ten days in the hospital, doctors told us, then at least three months in a brace. For those three months and longer, there are strict rules to follow: no riding in cars, no long periods of sitting. About 80 to 90 percent of the operations are successful; in others, the wobbliness of the spine still is not corrected.

What is ankylosis? This is fusion of two joints that occurs naturally, not by surgery. The stiffening occurs spontaneously.

What is a lumbar puncture? This is not an operation, but a testing and treatment procedure. Lumbar puncture is performed with a needle to measure the pressure of the cerebrospinal fluid, to withdraw some of the fluid for examination, or to introduce therapeutic or anesthetic agents into the space surrounding the spinal cord. The lumbar (low back) region is usually used because the space that surrounds the nerve roots there is large. Having the patient flex the trunk increases the space between the vertebrae. The needle is inserted in the skin a half inch from the midline to make an injection or remove fluid. When a spinal anesthetic is injected, the area of the body anesthetized may be controlled by the position of the patient.

How do you know what kind of operation is needed? You will have to rely on the judgment of your doctors, calling in specialists for second opinions when desirable. Many factors are involved in determining whether an operation will be effective and which one will be best. For example, only when there is spinal instability and when motion aggravates pain is fusion likely to help a patient.

Do you still need to do exercises if you have surgery? Yes. A good exercise program to strengthen the back is usually necessary before surgery and after surgery if the back is ever going to return to normal function and strength. But even better, many surgeons find that if the patient diligently follows a good exercise program like the one in this book, the back becomes so much better that surgery often is not necessary. Check with your doctor.

TOTAL HIP REPLACEMENT FOR ADOLESCENTS

Implanting artificial hips and hip joints was previously frowned upon for patients under sixty, but now total hip replacement is sometimes done in adolescents. Dr. Bernard H. Singsen, of the University of Southern California, reported on total hip replacements in children aged twelve to eighteen, who had either juvenile rheumatoid arthritis or ankylosing spondylitis. Before surgery, they had severe pain and deformity, and many were unable to walk. After the operation, all had complete relief of pain, and almost all achieved some or total ability to walk. At least a year of intense exercising and physical therapy is needed after surgery.

BONE GRAFTS FROM CADAVERS

Bone grafts for fusion operations on the spine used to be taken from a bone somewhere else in the patient's body, necessitating a more complicated operation. Now doctors can use bone from the legs of cadavers for a better graft, saving the patient a second operation, according to Dr. Theodore I. Malinin, of the University of Miami School of Medicine, Florida. If you sign papers to donate your eyes to an eye bank when you die, you can also designate that bones and other tissues can be used to help others.

HOW TO JUDGE A SURGEON

• Make sure he is "board certified" in his specialty. This means he has taken several years of specialty training after medical school, has at least two years' experience, and has passed an examination.

• Check his reputation with other doctors and nurses whom you know.

• Find out how frequently he does the particular operation you need done. You do not want a surgeon who does the operation only occasionally.

• Make sure he is on the staff at a good accredited hospital, preferably one that is a research or teaching institution or is affiliated with a medical school.

WHAT TO DO TO AVOID UNNECESSARY SURGERY

Don't go directly to a surgeon for medical treatment. A surgeon is more likely to suggest surgery than some other form of treatment. Your first visit should be to an internist or family practitioner, who will refer you to a surgeon if he thinks an operation may be needed.

When surgery is recommended, if there is any question of the need, obtain an independent opinion from another qualified surgeon.

Have your family doctor *and* your surgeon explain the alternatives to surgery, and both the benefits and possible complications of the alternatives and of the operation.

Don't push a doctor into performing surgery if he does not think it is needed.

Note: Blue Cross and other health plans in several states have announced that they will offer subscribers the opportunity to obtain a second professional opinion before undergoing non-emergency surgery. All charges related to the second opinion—the doctor's fee and the costs of X-rays or laboratory tests—will be paid for by the insurance plan.

WHAT TO DO BEFORE AND AT THE HOSPITAL TO REDUCE COMPLICATIONS AND TO RECOVER FASTER

If you are a smoker, stop smoking several days before surgery.

If you usually drink large amounts of alcohol, cut down before entering the hospital.

If you have had a cold or other respiratory infection recently, postpone elective surgery.

Loose or infected teeth should be removed if there is time.

Have plenty of rest and nourishing foods for the weeks preceding an operation.

Check with your doctor on muscle-strengthening exercises to do for the weeks before surgery.

Discuss with your doctor any chronic disease, allergies, or any medicine you take. He may want to adjust the dosage of some medications before surgery. If you have a chronic disease, have been taking cortisone or ACTH, are allergic to penicillin or other drugs, or if you have sickle cell anemia or other blood problems, you should inform both the anesthesiologist and the surgeon.

Take zinc tablets. Studies show that zinc sulfate makes wounds heal better and faster and with fewer complications.

Take vitamins. Several vitamins, such as A and C, also speed healing, so take high-strength vitamin and mineral tablets before surgery and during the recovery period.

Move around and exercise. Even in bed you can contract your feet and leg muscles. Sit up and walk as soon as your doctor says you can. This will not only help you heal faster, but will also help prevent dangerous blood clots from forming in the leg veins.

Yawn. Yawning helps inflate the lungs postoperatively, helping to clear bronchial secretions and prevent the pulmonary complications that often occur after surgery. Yawn five deep yawns every hour for the first five postoperative days.

IF YOU HAVE DIFFICULTY WITH FRACTURES HEALING

A Belgian physician has found that many cases of incomplete fracture healing are due to a deficiency of vitamin K. Bones of animals deficient in vitamin K were slow to heal; those given vitamin K healed promptly.

Other physicians use mild electric current to help fractures heal. Developed at the University of Pennsylvania, this technique involves putting an electrode at the fracture site and applying continuous, low-amperage current. So far, the cure rate has been better than 80 percent, often resulting in healing of fractures that have not healed in years. In some cases, bone pins are used as electrodes to carry the stimulating current; in others the process is completely external, using induction coils placed on the skin to apply the current.

A variation of this technique is just now being tested at Columbia University, using pulsating electromagnetic fields set up by coils right on the patient's cast. The technique has been used on more than 100 patients now with an 85 percent success rate in fractures that formerly were not healing.

GETTING ALONG WITH YOUR DOCTOR IN THE HOSPITAL

Doctors' visits in the hospital are brief because there are usually many patients to be seen, so make these visits as productive as possible. Prepare a list of questions or comments to present to your doctor when he stops by your room each day, and write down the significant things told to you.

You are now legally allowed to see your chart and can have access to all your medical records, but chances are you won't understand the medical terminology and abbreviations or even be able to read the handwriting, so ask your doctor to explain procedures, lab results, and medicines to you. This also gives you an extra check on medications to help ensure against the mistakes that occasionally happen even in the best of hospitals.

HOW TO PREVENT AND TREAT BEDSORES

Nasty ulcers of the skin can occur in bedridden patients when points of their body are in constant contact with the bed. To help prevent them, see that any bedridden patient is turned at two-hour intervals to a new position. Use a water or gel mattress. (Medicare will pay for its purchase or rental.)

Treatments. Laser beams are producing excellent results, says Dr. Eugene Seymour of Los Angeles, director of a referral center for laser treatment.

Dr. James W. Barnes, Jr., of Glenn Dale, Maryland, reports that packing the ulcer with sugar, then covering it with a thick, airtight dressing, produces healing in about 80 percent of cases. Dr. Robert Blomfield of Chelsea, England, reports in the *Journal of the American Medical Association* that honey used the same way is also effective. The honey was applied every two or three days under a dry dressing.

Dr. Thomas Coyle, rehabilitation specialist of Bridgeport, Connecticut, recommends a simple version of a water bed—an ordinary air mattress filled with warm water and kept warm with an electric blanket. Ulcers heal three times faster than usual with the warm water mattresses, he says, and, if used before bedsores develop, will often prevent them completely.

Dr. T. V. Taylor, of the University Hospital of South Manchester in England, reports that large doses of vitamin C resulted in twice as good healing in patients with bedsores compared to those who did not receive vitamin C supplements. The patients were given 500 milligrams of vitamin C twice a day.

Several studies indicate that zinc, both applied locally and taken as a dietary supplement, is of benefit to healing. Other doctors recommend that vitamin A and B vitamins, as well as adequate amounts of protein, also be added to the diet.

MAKING A BEDRIDDEN PATIENT MORE COMFORTABLE

• For a backrest, use a chair turned around, a campstool, or a board with a pillow propped in front of it.
• Place a box at the foot of the bed to prop the feet against.
• To take weight of bedclothes off feet, put a pillow at your feet and drape sheets and blankets over it.

TO PREVENT CONVALESCENT WOBBLY KNEES

Many people find their legs so weak after being bedridden that they can barely stand or walk. To avoid this, do these exercises while you're still in bed.

1. Keep your heel on the bed and shrug the kneecap by trying to draw it up. Do 8 to 10 times every hour whenever you are awake.

2. Stiffen and raise your leg off the bed. Do each leg 8 to 10 times per hour.

When you are allowed to sit up, sit on the edge of the bed with your legs dangling. Then extend your leg straight out. Repeat several times a day until fatigued.

IF YOU NEED NURSING HELP

Ask your doctor or his nurse for recommendations.

Call your local Visiting Nurse Association, the nursing department at your local hospital, or nurse registries in the yellow pages.

Have a cleaning woman or mother's helper take over the household chores while family members do the nursing.

You can have a nurse live in full-time, come in for eight hours a day, or come in as a visiting nurse, simply stopping by to check and give any necessary medications or advice.

Check for insurance coverage on nursing care.

R.N.   A registered nurse. Probably has gone to college or taken a four-year nursing course in a hospital. Licensed to administer medications and treatments.

L.P.N. A licensed practical nurse. Has had a shorter training period and in most states cannot administer medications unless supervised.

34 Pain that Doesn't Go Away and Drugless Ways to Treat It

The relentless pain of back problems sometimes doesn't seem to respond to any ordinary treatments. It goes on and on until the person's life seems centered around an unrelenting, burning, throbbing core of pain.

One report estimates that the average chronic-pain patient has suffered for seven years, undergone from three to five major operations, and spent from $50,000 to $100,000 in doctors' bills. In between the operations, he has taken countless drugs—from tranquilizers and muscle relaxants to potent narcotics—and there is at least a 50–50 chance that he has acquired a drug habit along the way.

But there are still things that can be done—new nonchemical techniques such as biofeedback, self-hypnosis, behavior modification, and ways of blocking nerve impulses that are proving effective for pain control when all other methods have failed.

Only in recent years has this kind of pain and pain treatment begun to get major scientific study, according to Dr. B. Berthold Wolff, chief of the Pain Study Group at New York University Medical School, and president of the newly organized American Pain Society. In fact, the treatment of chronic pain has developed into a new medical specialty called dolorology.

"Drugless ways of controlling pain are still considered to be on the oddball fringes of medicine," Dr. Wolff says, "but they very often work."

He recommended the newer, drugless treatment techniques at the latest national convention of the Arthritis Foundation.

Dr. Wolff stresses that the best results are often obtained with a combination of any two procedures.

BIOFEEDBACK

Biofeedback is a way to learn to control body functions that usually happen automatically. You work in a laboratory with a machine that lets you monitor the body functions you are interested in so you can begin to learn to control them.

You see your body functions on a TV-like screen. One screen might show finger temperature. If your muscles are tense, you might see an orange dot bob to the top of the screen. If your muscles are loose, the dot sinks to the bottom of the screen. By learning what keeps the dot near the bottom of the screen, you can learn to relax—or to help eradicate pain, even though you may not know exactly what you are doing.

"Imagine putting a golf ball," says Dr. Redford B. Williams, director of the new Clinical Biofeedback Laboratory at Duke University Medical Center. "After each putt, you adjust your swing until you get the ball in the hole. You'll never learn to putt if you can't see whether the ball goes to the left of the hole or to the right. Biofeedback training works much the same way. Instead of learning how to putt, a person can learn how to control his heartbeat or muscle tension."

Dr. Elmer E. Green, director of the Voluntary Controls Program at the Menninger Foundation in Topeka, Kansas, has been conducting research on biofeedback training since 1965. "When a doctor says your problem is that you are too tense, it doesn't help much," says Dr. Green. "But if a person can see his tension, then he can learn to manipulate it."

In many large cities, biofeedback laboratories are open to the public, and are even listed in the yellow pages; in other cities, persons must be referred by a psychologist or physician. Your physician should know if there is a center in your area. In addition to being used to counteract back pain, the biofeedback technique has proved especially effective in fighting stress and in treating headache, high blood pressure, Raynaud's disease, insomnia, phobias, heart arrhythmias, and speech problems.

SELF-HYPNOSIS

Whether you work from a commercially purchased tape or obtain instructions from your doctor, self-hypnosis can help you tolerate pain. It does not cure the source of the pain, but it makes you feel it less.

Dr. Herbert Spiegel, of New York's Columbia University College of Physicians and Surgeons, has taught a victim of whiplash pain to practice self-hypnosis whenever she has an attack. As she puts it: "I say to myself, 'It floats,' and the pain kind of dissipates. It's like turning down the volume on the radio."

Health writer Mark Bricklin uses self-hypnosis. First you get relaxed, he says, then you give yourself a very specific message. "It should be framed in positive terms. You don't tell yourself that you're not going to do this or that. Rather, you visualize yourself in the state you want to be in."

But you have to be careful not to overdo activity if you have eradicated pain, he says, once having done that himself after back strain, then waking up with a worse pain than ever. "What I should have done," he says, "was to numb the pain and then behave sensibly, letting my strained back muscles slowly return to normal."

TNS

The transcutaneous nerve stimulator is a new device that puts out low electric current to stimulate the skin at traditional acupuncture sites to relieve pain. A small stimulator, powered by two flashlight batteries, is worn by the patient at the appropriate location. For patients with arthritis of the hip, for example, the device is attached at waist level. The patient is taught to turn the TNS on as required, sometimes a dozen times a day. Periods of stimulation vary from fifteen minutes to two hours. The amplitude and frequency of the impulses can be controlled by two dials as desired, according to what works best for the pain. The patient feels a strong tingling.

The machine costs about $300 to $350 and is sometimes but not always covered by insurance. Patients are taught to use the device by a specially trained physician or physical therapist. Probably the most famous patient to use one was Alabama's Governor George Wallace.

Dr. Ronald Dougherty, medical director of Crouse Irving Memorial Hospital Pain Rehabilitation Clinic in Syracuse, New York, has treated patients with TNS combined with standard acupuncture. Of 100 patients with bursitis, arthritis, migraine, low back pain, or other chronic pain, 88 percent had relief of pain, he reports. Previously they had been addicted to drugs because of the severity of their pain. The traditional acupuncture treatment was given on an out-patient basis once a week at the hospital. And patients were given TNS units to use at home for up to four hours a day.

Dr. Ross Davis, neurosurgeon at Veterans Administration Hospital in Miami, Florida, who equipped Governor Wallace with his unit, says about 50 percent of spinal cord injury patients have had such relief of pain that they could stop medication. Another 10 to 20 percent have had some relief.

IMPLANTS

Just as TNS units can be used on the skin to give electric stimulation, special units can be permanently implanted to give out stimulation and deaden pain on command. At Sister Kenny Institute in Minneapolis, 170 such devices have been surgically placed, with a 60 percent success rate. The device is implanted in or near the spinal cord, with wires running under the skin to a tiny radio receiver on the chest. The patient activates the system with a battery-operated transmitter strapped to the waist. Impulses block the pain signals going to the brain.

Dr. John E. Adams, neurosurgeon of San Francisco, and Dr. Donald E. Richardson, of New Orleans, are implanting electrostimulators directly in the brain to switch off pain impulses. Relief of pain occurs in 50 to 75 percent of patients, they say.

CORDOTOMY

One of the oldest ways of dealing with chronic pain is surgery to cut pain-bearing nerve fibers. In a cordotomy, the sensory spinal nerves are cut or cauterized. Because motor-nerve fibers run parallel to the sensory ones, there are real risks of muscular weakness and even paralysis from the operation. And since the pain-relieving effects of a cordotomy frequently wear off after a year or two, the operation is usually reserved for terminal cancer patients.

Dr. Norman Shealy, of the Pain Rehabilitation Center in La Crosse, Wisconsin, warns against cordotomies. "The results are horrendous. They usually report complications of leg weakness in 5 to 10 percent and bladder problems in an equal amount; almost 100 percent of the patients are left with total or near total sexual impotence."

PERCUTANEOUS CORDOTOMY

This is a relatively new procedure for destroying certain nerve fibers in the spinal cord that carry pain impulses to the brain. It is done in about twenty minutes under local anesthesia, with the patient reporting during the operation what he feels. No knife is used, but a needle is placed between the first and second cervical vertebrae in the neck, and a radio-frequency current is applied through the needle to destroy the pain-carrying nerve fibers. Pain usually disappears completely, and the patient is able to return to work within a few weeks.

Dr. Hubert L. Rosomoff, chairman of the department of neurosurgery at the University of Miami (Florida) School of Medicine, one of the developers of the technique, has used it in more than 1,000 patients.

Dr. Rosomoff explains that the operation can be done because pain sensations from all over the body go up separate nerve fibers from other sensations, and so can be destroyed where they are separated out in the neck part of the spinal cord.

The entry of the needle is watched via a special X-ray TV unit where the doctor can see the needle enter the spinal canal. A thin wire is then guided through the needle until it reaches the correct spot in the spinal cord. It serves as the electrode for the nerve-destroying current. Short bursts of current are given until the patient describes relief of pain during the operation. Sometimes, he said, patients actually burst into tears of relief on the operating table, as, for the first time in months, their pain disappears.

There is a 1 to 2 percent chance of side effects from the procedure, sometimes a temporary weakness on one side of the body, difficulty in breathing, or the eyelid may droop for a short time. One permanent side effect is that patients will not be able to feel hot or cold. Some patients are said to be left with sexual impotence. About 10 percent are said to develop a burning pain.

Percutaneous cordotomy appears to give relief to about 80 percent of patients. Some patients need the procedure done more than once.

PAIN CLINICS

If you have serious long-lasting pain that cannot seem to be helped by ordinary medical measures, there are specialized pain clinics that have recently been established in a number of medical centers to deal with this problem. Techniques they use include neurosurgery, electrical stimulation, hypnosis, nerve blocks, biofeedback, muscle relaxation training, spinal injections, dietary instruction, acupuncture, psychotherapy, physical therapy, and drug withdrawal.

Some treatments are done while you're in the hospital, others are on an out-patient basis.

One typical pain clinic program is the one at the University of Washington. The patient is examined by specialists in several fields: anesthesiology, general surgery, internal medicine, neurology, neurosurgery, nursing, oral surgery, orthopedics, pharmacology, physiatry, psychiatry, psychology, radiology, and sociology. At a weekly conference, the entire specialty team considers the patient's pain problem and works out a program of therapy. A patient manager coordinates therapy until the patient can be sent back to his referring physician for continuation of treatment.

At the Pain Rehabilitation Center, in La Crosse, Wisconsin, there is even more of a holistic approach, with nearly every possible treatment offered that has any potential benefit. There, at a clinic located on a farm, not only are rest, heat, ice, massage, physiotherapy, exercises, behavior modification, and counseling given, but also percutaneous electrical stimulation, acupuncture, biofeedback, implants, the new surgical technique of facet degeneration, and diet.

"We flood our patients with vitamins in supertherapeutic dosages since many of them are not in very good physical condition anyway," says director Dr. C. Norman Shealy. He also encourages patients to avoid sugar, hydrogenated oils and fats (using butter, pork lard, or vegetable cooking oils instead), food additives and all processed foods, tobacco and caffeine and to limit alcohol to no more than two ounces a day.

The twelve-day program, including room, meals, and all medical therapy, averages about $1,500.

"At this point," says Shealy," it appears that 64 percent of our patients remain in good or excellent condition six months later. About 25 to 30 percent return to work." Getting the patients off drugs and out of the pain game is doing a tremendous job in saving society money, he says.

WHAT TO EXPECT IN A PAIN TREATMENT CENTER

The Johns Hopkins Pain Treatment Center is a typical one. It was begun for people with chronic pain problems unresolved by usual types of medical care. It incorporates standard treatments for pain as well as most of the newest approaches. The primary objective is to eliminate or significantly reduce pain and, when that's impossible, to help the patient learn to tolerate the disability and to return to a more normal, productive life.

Some fortunate individuals require only a short time to obtain relief, a spokesman said. "But it is wise to plan on a two-week stay or longer."

Goals are set for each patient—a treatment goal, an occupational goal, and a family or personal relationship goal. Each patient carefully formulates his own goals with the staff during hospitalization.

"Much of the treatment will be different than anything you have experienced in a hospital previously, and your relationship with the physicians and other members of the professional staff will also be different than the traditional patient-doctor relationship," I was told.

Patients may be referred by any physician, rehabilitation agencies, insurance agencies, or themselves. There is often a five-month waiting list. Complete records from doctors who have been involved in your treatment and X-rays must be sent.

Before admission, each patient completes a questionnaire with information on his pain problem. On admission you are examined and your case is reviewed by members of the nursing and medical staffs. The cause of your pain will be determined, if possible, and appropriate treatments outlined.

The pain treatment program has three basic aims. The first is relief of pain if possible. The second is elimination of all, or nearly all, drugs from daily life, including all kinds of narcotic pain relievers, most kinds of sleeping pills, and most tranquilizers. The third aim is to increase each patient's activity level to the point that they can again become useful family or society members.

The major technique used is electrical stimulation to block pain—the TNS stimulator applied to the skin on and around the painful area. This trial usually takes one to three days to see if it is effective. If not effective, the next step normally is to apply stimulation directly to a nerve by means of needles placed through the skin. If this is not effective and the pain is severe, actual stimulation of the spinal cord, or the nerves where they branch off the spinal cord, may be used.

Other techniques include biofeedback, nerve blocks, acupuncture, and implants of electrical stimulators.

There is a graded program to eliminate as many drugs as possible after treatment has begun. Drug misuse, abuse, or frank addiction are extremely common in patients suffering from chronic pain, I was told. Drugs are given only on schedule. You are not allowed to ask the nurse for additional medication, and you can obtain medication only when the schedule calls for drugs to be administered.

"A firm conviction that you want to be free of the need for drugs is the basic requirement of our pain treatment program," I was told. "You must wish to stop all of these harmful drugs or it is useless to enter the pain treatment program. If you decide you cannot do without them, ask to be discharged from the program. If you take drugs on your own without our permission, you will be discharged from the program."

The program includes an assessment of such simple things as walking, stair climbing, sitting, standing, reclining, and other activities, and a graded program to try to bring them to near normal. You are instructed in therapeutic exercises. Once it has been determined that your activity level will not worsen your disease state, you may be asked to do exercises in spite of discomfort.

The patient is asked not to discuss his pain with other patients, family, or visitors. "We wish to encourage the patients to think about positive aspects of life," I was told. "We specifically do not wish patients to discuss their various pains among themselves. Any patient who continues to do so, or to exhibit complaints of pain and pain behavior in spite of these instructions, may be asked to leave."

"This program is simply a beginning for a new way of life," the spokesman said. "It is expected that all of the principles and treatments utilized here will be continued on an on-going basis when the patient returns home. This is not an easy program for the professional staff or for the patient. However, if you have a sincere desire to be pain-free, to resume a more normal life, and to eliminate the regular use of drugs, the program has an excellent chance of helping you."

MAJOR U.S. PAIN CLINICS

The following clinics specialize in treatment of pain. Most of them require that the patient be referred to them by a doctor.

Pain Center, City of Hope National Medical Center, 1500 East Duarte Road, Duarte, California 91010.

Pain Treatment Center, Hospital of Scripps Clinic, 10660 North Tarry Anis Road, La Jolla, California 92037.

UCLA Pain Management Clinic, UCLA School of Medicine, 10833 Le Conte Avenue, Los Angeles, California 90024.

Pain Center, Mount Zion Hospital and Medical Center, 1600 Divisadero Street, San Francisco, California 94115.

Portland Pain Rehabilitation Center, Emmanuel Hospital, 3001 North Gantenbein Avenue, Portland, Oregon 97227.

Pain Clinic, Georgetown Medical Center, Washington, D.C. 20007.

Pain & Health Rehabilitation Center, Route 2, Welsh Coulee, La Crosse, Wisconsin 54601.

Pain Clinic, University of Washington School of Medicine, Seattle, Washington 98195.

Pain Center, Rush Medical College, Rush-Presbyterian-St. Luke's Medical Center, 1725 Harrison Street, Chicago, Illinois 60612.

Pain Clinic, University of Illinois College of Medicine, 840 South Wood Street, Chicago, Illinois 60612.

Pain Management Center, Mayo Clinic–St. Mary's Hospital of Rochester, Rochester, Minnesota 55901.

Pain Unit, Massachusetts Rehabilitation Hospital, 125 Nashua Street, Boston, Massachusetts 02114.

Nebraska Pain Rehabilitation Unit, University of Nebraska College of Medicine, Omaha, Nebraska 68105.

The Center, Mesa Lutheran Hospital, 525 West Crown Road, Mesa, Arizona 85201.

Pain Consultation Center, Mount Sinai Medical Center, 4300 Alton Road, Miami Beach, Florida 33140.

Pain Clinic, Johns Hopkins University School of Medicine, Baltimore, Maryland 21205.

Nerve Block and Pain Studies Clinic, University of Virginia Medical Center, Charlottesville, Virginia 22903.

35 The Pain Game

Many people with chronic back pain are playing pain games, doctors told me. Such patients seem to obtain enough benefit from the pain to want to continue it. Their pain becomes the focus of their life. They become addicted to the attention and sympathy from others, and find they are often catered to by family and friends.

As Dr. Wilbert E. Fordyce, psychologist at the University of Washington School of Medicine, pointed out, when the back hurts, many people find it can set up a pattern for avoiding work, getting a pleasant high from a painkiller, or receiving attention and sympathy. He and other doctors use a kind of behavior modification called operant conditioning to help patients overcome their pain behavior. Praise and attention are given for activity and accomplishments rather than for pain. These methods now constitute a major part of most pain treatment programs. If action such as these procedures is not taken, Fordyce says, the pain behavior can lead to drug abuse, extreme inactivity, and other destructive life patterns.

"We are not being cynical when we use the term 'pain game' and do not wish to make light of chronic suffering," says Dr. C. Norman Shealy, director of the Pain and Health Treatment Center in La Crosse, Wisconsin. "There is nothing pleasurable or funny about it, as the misery of patients and the unhappiness of their families can testify.

"On the other hand, as long as the patient allows his suffering to govern his behavior, that is the 'game' he is playing, and there is little chance for relief." And sometimes, he says, what starts as a short game sometimes becomes a life script.

"Some patients build their life-style around their pain, enjoying poor health. . . . At the very least, pain behavior is like a mindless bad habit."

The cost to the back sufferer and to society is huge, he says. One chronic pain patient who came to him, Shealy said, was a man who had had forty operations with medical costs of $450,000. Only about 39 percent of Workmen's Compensation patients who have suffered back injuries return to work, he notes. And although the chronic pain sufferers represent a mere 2 or 3 percent of the total number of people injured at work, somewhere between 50 and 75 percent of the medical costs of Workmen's Compensation goes for their treatment.

The divorce rate for pain patients, too, is remarkably high— between 60 and 80 percent.

RECOGNIZING THE PAIN GAME

Dr. Richard A. Sternbach, director of the Pain Treatment Center at Scripps Clinic in La Jolla, California, says some patients are low back losers.

"The former ways of getting strokes and payoffs, and in general feeling good, are no longer available to them," says Sternbach. "Thus, if admiration used to come from being a productive worker, now it can only come from letting people know how much one suffers, yet tries to be brave."

The patients may need to keep their pain as a mark of suffering or proof of disability, says Sternbach. "Or they may have built up so much resentment toward doctors for continual referrals, tests, clinic visits, and hospital stays, with no pain relief, that they now must defeat the doctors." They confound the doctor by keeping their pain.

There is too much prescribing of tranquilizers, too, says Dr. Sternbach. There is an important difference between the anxious person with acute pain and the depressed patient with chronic pain, he says. In acute cases, treatment of anxiety by repeated reassurances and minor tranquilizers can reduce pain. But continued use of the anti-anxiety agents when the patient has passed into the chronic pain state can make the depression more severe. Depression is best treated by antidepressant medicine and by such rehabilitation maneuvers as increasing activity, vocational retraining, and giving reasons to be hopeful.

The patient does not appear depressed and usually denies any feelings of depression, Dr. Sternbach says, yet most patients are significantly depressed and have disturbances in sleep, appetite, libido, and general performance. And the patients are very preoccupied, over-concerned about symptoms.

Some patients with low back pain do have *some* physical symptoms, but not enough to account for the severity of complaints or to warrant repeated surgery, says Sternbach.

"These patients make a career of suffering and often attempt to defeat doctors' efforts to diagnose their pain and relieve their suffering. For example, when saying to our low back patients: 'It looks as though the doctors can't help you,' instead of tears or looks of desperation, we often observe tight smiles of satisfaction."

Other signs of the low back pain game: Multiple operations without relief of pain, giving up work, having a dependent relationship at home, or playing "Yes, but . . ." games with the doctor.

WHAT TO DO TO GET OUT OF THE PAIN GAME

Set goals. As a rule of thumb, says Sternbach, the patient who has clear-cut goals and begins to work at them will have a better treatment outcome than one who has no such goals.

In pain treatment or rehabilitation, as in much else, motivation is crucial, he observes.

"Progress toward goals should be broken up into units of time which are short enough that the patient can readily perceive any progress," he says. For example, if the patient wishes to be able to sit long enough to join his friends for a four-hour card game each week, and if his tolerance for sitting is one hour, at which point pain increases, then every evening he can sit at home to play solitaire for forty-five minutes for several days, then gradually increase the time by ten minutes until he reaches his goal. The same can be done for walking and other activities. The meeting of the quota is a positive reinforcement because the patient can see his progress.

The patient must have a clear set of reasons for getting better, says Sternbach. "Taking account of his disabilities, what would the patient do if the pain were eliminated? Specifically, what would he do for fun or money or to meet his social needs? As life becomes more satisfying and his depression lifts, the severity and number of his complaints tend to decrease."

Get help with depression and with coping. Dr. J. Blair Pace, at a back clinic in Downey, California, says that often when he treats a back patient for his or her depression, the back pain goes away. In fact, he says he has cured more chronic low back pain with antidepressants than with any other treatment.

In *Emergency Medicine* he described to other doctors typical conversations he has with patients who are not handling their back pain well. He says he tells patients such things as "Look, we know you hurt. All this pain is real but your pain seems to be greatly exaggerated by the fact that you're very worried." Or: "Your life situation is so painful that you use the physical pain to cope with it. Why don't we try looking for another way of coping?"

Dr. Pace also asks patients to design specific goals for themselves—to lose weight or to walk twice as far next week as this week, and so on.

Dr. Jack J. Pinsky, associate director of the City of Hope Pain Center in Duarte, California, reports success with patients using group psychotherapy sessions. Patients responded unexpectedly well to an intense sixty hours of therapy over seven weeks, he said.

Don't get dependent on Workmen's Compensation. Workmen's Comp is often a part of the pain game. Dr. Steven F. Brena, director of the Emory University Pain Control Center in Atlanta, Georgia, cites an Emory experiment in which patients receiving financial compensation for work-related injuries were compared with a similar group receiving no compensation but with the same degree of organic disease. The patients who received payments were significantly less likely to show improvement, were less likely to follow programmed instructions, and had a higher dropout rate.

Get up and get moving. Dr. Shealy says at their center in La Crosse nurses are taught not to pamper the patients but to urge them into physical activities. Patients are assigned walking to do every day, varying from about one half of a city block up to five city blocks. They are further required to ride a stationary bicycle or a movable one, adding one minute per day to their time, and to go to the swimming pool five days a week for an hour. Special limbering exercises are also done twice a day.

Many of his patients find, to their delight, that they can be much more active than they had realized, says Shealy. "One patient recently hobbled into the clinic with a cane, claiming that he could hardly take five steps without it. On the third day in our program, he walked five *blocks* to and from a restaurant—without his cane!"

In most cases, Dr. Sternbach adds, the exercising not only results in a markedly improved range of motion, but also improves patients' self-image, since it is difficult for those who spend several hours daily in physical activity to sustain the picture of being a chronic invalid.

Get your family into the act. Discuss with them, and have your doctor talk to them about the behavior modification techniques we have discussed in this book that are used in pain centers. Let your family and close friends know you sincerely want to begin to stop thinking of pain and start expanding your life.

Dr. Pace says he frequently works with families. "For instance, we tell a daughter: 'Your mother uses her pain to get your attention. Give her lots of attention for anything except the complaint of pain.' The family has to learn to react this way in order to change the patient's behavioral pattern."

Even if pain is not completely eliminated, he says, the patient has an entirely different outlook and can return to an active life.

HOW TO BREAK THE DRUG HABIT

Taking drugs is perhaps the most insidious of all the pain patient's conditioned habits, according to Dr. Shealy. "Drugs almost invariably alter the patient's personality and decrease his physical activity. Yet they do not satisfactorily relieve his pain; instead, tolerance occurs within a few weeks, which makes higher and higher doses necessary."

Dr. Shealy uses several methods to help patients break the drug habit. All medication is packaged in capsules of the same size, shape, and color, so it is not difficult to change the drug dosage or to switch the drug to a safer one without the patient's knowledge. All tranquilizers and sedatives are converted to sodium amytal. Strong antidepressants are converted to Elavil taken at bedtime. Narcotics are converted to methadone. Strong painkillers are converted to aspirin or Tylenol. Also Shealy says all medications at his center are given on a time schedule established by the doctor and are not given whenever the patient thinks he needs them. The dosages of these drugs are gradually reduced, he says, over a one- to two-week period.

"When the patient's drug dosage has been reduced to nothing and he has actually been taking a placebo for several days, he is made aware of that fact, and almost invariably patients will admit that their pain is no worse!"

PATIENT-DOCTOR GROUND RULES

Patients tend to become frustrated with their physicians, and physicians often become exasperated with patients, says Dr. Sternbach. To avoid such difficulties it may be helpful to spell out some ground rules and rights to which both parties can agree.

For example, he says, the patient has the right to a once or twice yearly reevaluation of his pain problem without being made to feel like a hypochondriac. On the other hand, the physician has the right to be spared "urgent" calls and visits. Chronic pain is seldom an emergency. (An exception is made for the sudden appearance of a new and different pain.)

The patient has a right to be informed of new developments related to his problem, which may give him reason to be hopeful, without having to pry them out of his doctor. The physician has the right to expect the patient to follow through on physical therapy, weight control, vocational rehabilitation, pacing activities, and self-control in medication usage.

The patient has the right to tell his doctor about personal and psychological problems without having the physician reject these issues as irrelevant. The physician has the right to recommend psychological or psychiatric intervention without having the patient be insulted.

36 How to Get the Most from Your Health Insurance Dollar

Four out of five Americans with back problems have health insurance of some kind. But they often find out—too late—that their insurance usually covers less than they thought, or perhaps doesn't cover their problem at all.

CHECK WHAT KIND OF INSURANCE YOU HAVE

Hospital expense insurance. This pays all or part of the cost of hospital room, board, X-rays, medicines, and other expenses in the hospital. Some plans reimburse the patient. Others pay the hospital directly.

Surgical expense insurance. This pays part or all of the cost of an operation. The amount depends on the nature of the operation.

Medical expense insurance. Under this plan, visits to a doctor's office or his house calls are reimbursed according to a limit set in the policy.

Major Medical expense insurance. This insurance helps to pay the cost of extended sickness or injury. The policies generally have a deductible clause; typically, the patient pays the first $100 or $200 himself, then the plan pays 80 percent of the balance, up to some limit, perhaps $100,000.

Loss-of-income insurance. This insurance, also called Disability Income Insurance, pays benefits when the insured person is unable to work because of illness or injury.

Prepaid group health plan. In these plans, like Kaiser-Permanente, you pay a yearly fee to a group of health specialists for regular checkups and treatment, and sometimes for stays in a hospital.

Cooperatives. A cooperative is operated by a board of directors chosen from its own membership, which contracts with a medical staff for provision of services on a salary rather than on a fee-for-service basis.

Health maintenance organization. This is comprehensive medical care, with emphasis on preventive and maintenance medicine to try to keep the patient healthy and out of the hospital. The idea of HMOs is to collect fees to keep people well instead of to cure them after they're sick.

NINE CHECKPOINTS THAT COULD SAVE YOU MONEY

Check your benefits. A lot of people don't use the insurance they have, and actually pay medical bills themselves when they are covered by insurance. On the other hand, you may not be covered for something for which you think you are insured. Check with your agent and ask about any fine print you don't understand.

Don't have elective surgery until you read your policy. Before you schedule surgery, check to see if your policy will be in effect. There also may be a waiting period before benefits are paid for treatment for a preexisting condition.

Check your doctor or hospital bill. Insist on knowing what charges are for. You may legitimately owe them or you may not.

Check for duplications of insurance. If both husband and wife work, there may be duplicate insurance coverage. If you do have overlapping policies and one pays you directly instead of the hospital, it is sometimes possible to collect from both policies.

Avoid overly expensive hospital rooms. Many policies cover only a fixed amount for a hospital room, no matter what the actual room rate is. If your policy has a limit of $50 a day in a hospital and you're in a $150-a-day private room, you pay the difference.

Check your insurance policy for out-patient tests. Many insurance companies will pay for tests only if they are done in a hospital, a ridiculous waste of money and time, since many of the tests can be done in a few hours, and the patient dismissed. See what your policy covers.

Be sure you are collecting what you can from Medicare. Things keep changing under Medicare, so you may have different benefits now from when it first began.

Don't overlook the new benefits in your Social Security program. Under the disability provision, if a person becomes totally disabled and cannot work, he will be able to draw the same benefits immediately that he would have at retirement.

Check military benefits if you are eligible. The Civilian Health and Medical Program for the Uniformed Services (CHAMPUS) is available to dependents of servicemen, retired servicemen, and the dependents of deceased servicemen. The benefits also apply to the National Oceanic and Atmospheric Association and the Commissioned Corps of the Public Health Service. Millions are eligible to get treatment at civilian medical facilities, if it isn't conveniently available from the military, and have most of their bills paid. If you think you are eligible, contact your County Veteran Service Officer or CHAMPUS, Denver, Colorado 80240.

MEDICARE

Medicare is a program of health insurance under Social Security that helps those sixty-five and older pay for health care. Most people sixty-five and older are automatically eligible for the *hospital insurance,* which pays for care in a hospital. You can also sign up for *medical insurance,* which helps pay doctor bills and other medical items and services not covered under hospital insurance. The medical program is voluntary; no one is covered automatically.

If you are not certain whether you are eligible for either program, call any Social Security office for information.

To make sure you get the full protection of Medicare, starting with the month you reach sixty-five, you should sign up with your Social Security office at least a month before your birthday.

The benefits covered. Your *hospital insurance* will pay the cost of the room and meals in semiprivate accommodations (two to four beds), regular nursing services, drugs, supplies, and appliances. It will not pay for doctor bills, private duty nurses, telephone, or television.

The *medical insurance* part of Medicare helps pay for physicians' services given in the doctor's office, the hospital, or your home, as well as for out-patient hospital services in an emergency room or out-patient clinic. It does not cover routine physical checkups, orthopedic shoes, and services provided outside the United States.

Benefits are occasionally changed. You can call any Social Security office for more detailed information about the latest regulations.

Recommended. *Your Medicare Handbook,* a booklet explaining all phases of Medicare. U.S. Printing Office, Washington, D.C. 20402. 35 cents.

YOUR BACK AND THE IRS

Don't forget the medical deductions on your federal (and sometimes state and city) income taxes.

Here are some of the costs you can deduct from your income tax. The rules often change from year to year, but usually the following can be figured as part of your medical deduction.

Some medical insurance premiums.

Supplementary medical insurance under Medicare.

Payments to physicians, surgeons, chiropractors, osteopaths, chiropodists, podiatrists, psychiatrists, psychologists, and Christian Science practitioners.

Payments for hospital services, therapy, laboratory, surgical, obstetrical, X-ray, nursing services (including nurse's board paid by you), and ambulances.

Charges for medical care included in the tuition fee of a college or private school or retirement home.

Payments for psychiatric care.

A parent's transportation expenses for regular visits recommended as part of a child's therapy.

Payments for medicines and drugs and prescribed vitamins that exceed 1 percent of your adjusted gross income.

A special food or beverage prescribed by a physician for the treatment of an illness.

Payment for transportation essential to medical care, including bus, taxi, train or plane fares, parking fees (or 6 cents per mile if you use your car).

Meals and lodging that are a necessary part of medical care.

Payments for sending a mentally or physically handicapped child to a special school.

Payments for special equipment installed in a home or car for medical purposes.

Payment for artificial limbs and crutches.

WHAT TO DO IF YOU ARE HURT AT WORK.

I talked to David P. Karcher, an attorney in Miami who specializes in insurance and compensation cases. He gives the following advice.

Once the emergency or medical treatment is taken care of, call your supervisor or the medical department where you work to confirm that they know what has happened to you and that proper procedures have been begun by them for handling your work and for processing the appropriate medical insurance forms. In most cases procedures are handled routinely and pretty much automatically. Your employer makes a report to the insurance company. Your doctor fills out a report form and submits a bill to the insurance company. The insurance company will usually send a letter or report letting you know how much you can personally expect in the way of payments from lost pay or for reimbursed money if you paid any medical bills yourself.

Payments are made for lost wages and medical bills without any problem within a few weeks in 85 percent of the cases, Karcher says.

In the 15 percent of cases where there is some dispute, he says to first discuss the situation with your boss and his insurance company and also have your physician talk with them to make sure they completely understand all the facts in the case. If a satisfactory solution still has not been found, he says, it is time to go to an attorney who handles insurance claims. If you don't know of any such attorney, contact your local bar association and ask them for the names of lawyers in your area who they recommend to specialize in Workmen's Compensation cases. (The bar association may be listed in the telephone book under the name of your city, county, or state, or under Lawyer Referral Service. Or now that the U.S. Supreme Court allows advertising by lawyers, you might find a lawyer listed in the yellow pages under "attorneys" or "lawyers," with his or her specialty indicated.)

What can you expect to get? The employer or the insurance company will usually pay for medical treatments until there is maximum medical improvement; in other words, until treatment isn't able to make you any better.

And they will pay all or part of lost wages, the amount differing with different employers and different states. A typical payment would be 60 percent of your usual weekly wage.

In addition to all or some of your lost wages and payment of medical bills, if you have any permanent disability from the injury that occurred at the job, you will probably be able to obtain an award for that, says Karcher. "Permanency" is based on the theoretical loss of wage-earning capacity, with slightly different interpretations in different states. In some states this means that if you were earning $100 before the injury and you went back to work afterward and got the same salary, there was no permanent disability of any kind. In other states, if the doctor says you have a 10 percent or whatever percent disability, you are paid for that, no matter what your returning salary level is.

The length of time varies for payment of this money. In Florida, for example, for permanent partial disability (P.P.D. the lawyers call it) the most you can be entitled to is payment for 350 weeks. If your doctor said you had a 10 percent disability, you would then receive payments for 10 percent of 350 weeks, or 35 weeks.

If you have total disability, you may be awarded compensation for the rest of your life.

If your employment comes under federal law, for example, if you are a longshoreman or shipbuilder, you would get two-thirds of the difference between your average weekly wage before and after the accident, assuming it was less afterward. You would receive this as long as the disability lasted, which might be forever.

What about cheating? There are many ways to catch the cheat, says Karcher. "There are certain patterns to numbness or pain that show whether damage is fake or real. And there are all kinds of tricks attorneys and doctors have, such as having the victim demonstrate the farthest they can turn their neck or back since the accident, then asking them how far they could turn before the accident. You'd be surprised at how many will show you!"

WHAT TO DO IF YOU ARE IN A CAR ACCIDENT

Have someone call the police, and an ambulance or doctor if needed.

Get the case number of the report from the police officer, and his name.

Exchange names, addresses, telephone numbers, license numbers, drivers license numbers, and names and phone numbers of insurance companies with all persons involved.

Go to a hospital or see a physician for an examination, even though injuries may seem minor.

Call your insurance company and give your agent all the information. Also report the accident to the other person's insurance company.

Get a copy of the police officer's report from the police station.

An adjuster will come and talk to you. If you are happy with their offer of payment, take it.

If you think it isn't fair or that you are entitled to more, or if you feel that the true extent of your injuries is not yet really determined, don't sign any release forms. (Things often develop days or weeks later, especially when the neck or back is involved.)

It should only be necessary to consult a lawyer to start a lawsuit if you consider the insurance company's offer to be unfair or inadequate.

HOW YOUR DOCTOR CAN HELP SAVE YOUR JOB

It's harder to find a new job than it is to keep the old one. And how you do at getting back to your job after a back injury can be partly up to your doctor, says Dr. George E. Ehrlich, professor of rehabilitation medicine at Temple University School of Medicine.

"I've found that if the doctor discusses the problem with an employer at the beginning, the employer usually is willing to go along with the treatment program in the interest of keeping a good employee," says Dr. Ehrlich.

Here are some things he says you can have your doctor do to keep your employer on your side and help have your job still waiting for you when your back is healed.

Have your doctor let your employer know immediately what the diagnosis is (often he must have your permission to do this).

Have him keep your employer informed about your progress since he can best answer questions your employer may ask and can convince the employer more effectively that you are truly making progress toward recovery.

Have him explain, if your condition will take quite a while to heal, that you will probably have to take some time off during the next six months or whatever time, but that afterwards you may well be able to do the same good job as before.

Have him assure your employer that there will not be any increase in the insurance rate, which he can confirm with his insurance company.

If your employer is not willing to keep you on, have your doctor get in touch with your union right away, if you belong to one. "But act quickly," says Ehrlich. "The union will be more receptive about backing someone up while he's employed than when he's out of work."

If it turns out you won't be able to return to your old job because you end up with a permanent disability and simply can't function as well, have your doctor suggest that you wish to continue working and that you can be trained for some other type of work in the company.

Confirm to your doctor frequently that you do not want to fall unnecessarily into a dependent role, and that you want to get back to as full a function as possible in both your job and your family, that you want to be independent and productive.

COMPENSATIONITIS

Don't be guilty of compensationitis, says Dr. Eugene Nordby, of Madison, Wisconsin. That's an exaggerated reaction to an injury to gain more money or to keep from going back to a job that is not fulfilling.

It is a well-known fact that the fastest way to get persons well is to have their compensation settlement paid, he says. "We call it the greenback poultice." But this isn't always due to faking or malingering, says Dr. Nordby. Sometimes there are subconscious forces at work.

"One of the well-meaning fringe benefits that presents an insurmountable problem is that where there is no wage loss while disabled for work due to illness or injury that is compensable, what incentive is there to return to work?"

And sometimes there really is faking; then detective work must be brutal and is necessary, he says. "One such example involved a movie of a young man, allegedly completely disabled, playing in a vigorous basketball game.

"Frequently the cooperation of the employer in allowing an injured employee to return to part-time or lighter work can be most helpful in providing a therapeutic mechanism to give credence to the physical injury and bridge the gap in returning to regular work," he says. "Some insurance carriers have partial disability payments that help in this respect if the lighter job is less rewarding financially, even when pursued full-time."

That an unsettled claim for compensation can often tend to prolong pain and slow down recovery was mentioned by many doctors we talked to. The patient's wish to become well may unconsciously be outweighed by his fear of what will happen in the future and the security promised from compensation. In addition, his claims may be viewed with suspicion by doctor and employer so he feels he must prove his illness and pain. Once settlement is made, the pressure to remain ill is off the patient; his illness has been recognized and he can direct his energies to recovering.

Other doctors caution patients not to be upset about what they call post-traumatic neurosis, a common reaction to serious physical injury from an accident. When, often days or weeks later, the person suddenly realizes fully the threat to life and limb, the peril he or she has been through, it frequently causes a major personality upheaval for a time. He or she becomes anxious and irritable or incensed by the invasion of body and life by hidden perils. Police report the same type of reaction in people who have been assaulted or whose homes have been broken into, exposing them and their family to danger. Understanding that the reaction is common makes it easier for the victim and family to deal with it.

37 How to Give a Great Back Rub and Massage

A massage will not cure arthritis or sciatica or an injury, but it can make you feel better even if it does not cure the underlying problem. It can relax muscles, help relieve muscle spasms, increase circulation, and soothe taut nerves.

Different massage techniques are often used for different problems. If a person has a slipped disk and the muscles have contracted to protect the nerves, an easy stroking motion is usually used. To relax the entire body, especially the spine, the spinal column is massaged from the neck to the tailbone.

Massage treatment by a physical therapist often begins with an application of heat to the affected area to relax muscles that are taut or cramped. Hot towels are sometimes applied for moist superficial heat, or infrared lamps for a dry superficial heat. Occasionally diathermy machines are used for very deep heat penetration.

When treating a specific area, physical therapists usually work from the point closest to the heart outward. They don't work on the injured area immediately; for an injured ankle, for example, they would begin massaging the hip, then the thigh, the knee, the calf, and then move to the ankle.

Most commercial masseurs work in the opposite direction—from the legs and arms to the back and heart. For a general massage, both masseurs and physical therapists make their strokes toward the heart, to move the blood in the veins toward the heart.

In health spas, steam baths and saunas are often taken before a massage. There are two benefits: psychological relaxation and specific physical relaxation of muscles from the heat.

Are there any dangers? The American Medical Association says people with a heart or respiratory problem would do well to stay out of saunas. And they say people with varicose veins, arthritis, or diabetic neuritis should check with their doctor before having a massage. Otherwise they make you feel great.

SECRETS FROM THE PROFESSIONALS

Mineral or vegetable oil, talcum or body powder aid smoothness. The massage should be given on the floor with some padding, such as a foam mat or thick quilt. A bed usually is not firm enough.

Weight rather than muscle should be used to apply pressure.

If there is a tense spot, a wide area around it should be massaged first, then the tense spot should be massaged using strong pressure.

When you are receiving a massage, keep your body as limp as you can. Do not try to help. Let yourself be completely taken care of.

Strokes can be made with the palm, heel or edge of the hand, with just the fingers, or even with one finger or thumb, and can include the following: the hands slipping over the skin; the hands not slipping over the skin, but making the superficial skin tissue move over the deeper underlying tissue; light, slow, gentle stroking; deep stroking; lifting or kneading the tissue; rolling with the palms; raking the skin with the fingers; moving fingertips with deep pressure in tiny circles; large sweeps with the forearms; light slapping.

Strokes should be smooth and steady, never uneven or jerky.

The entire area of the body being massaged should be completely and systematically covered.

The massager should always try to have one hand touching you, without breaking contact once it is established.

The massager should let fingers and hands explore the inner anatomy of the area being massaged, feeling the shape and texture of the underlying bones and muscles and tissue structures.

THE BETTER BACK EXPERT BACK MASSAGE

Have subject lie face down, limp and loose. Cover the forehead with the fingers of both hands; stroke sideways toward the hairline. Massage the temples with the balls of the fingers. Stroke across the eyebrows to above the ears.

Slide the fingers to the middle of the head; slowly cover the entire scalp with firm circles. Work small circles down the midline of the neck, feeling the structure of bone and muscle beneath. Stroke down the outward neck muscles; make large circles at the base of the neck. Make several strokes out along the shoulders.

Gently turn the subject's head so it is resting sideways, on one cheek instead of face down.

Massage one hand, with small circles, first the back of the hand, then the heel, then the inside of the wrist. Grasp the thumb where it joins the hand and pull slowly from the base to the tip of the thumb, twisting gently back and forth. Do each finger in the same way.

Place both your hands around subject's wrist, and squeeze your way up the arm. Starting at the wrist again, stroke firmly in a milking motion to push the blood toward the body. Repeat on the other arm.

With the thumbs of both hands, massage the sole of one foot in small firm circles, then the top of the foot, then around the ankle. Twist and pull each toe as you did the fingers. Grasp the ankle with both hands, and massage in a milking motion up to the hip. Slide both hands back to the ankle. Repeat. Then starting again at the ankle, pull your hands upward, firmly pushing the blood toward the body as you did with the arms. Repeat the entire massage on the other foot and leg.

Using very light strokes, outline the buttocks, then knead the entire area of both buttocks as if you were kneading bread. Then place your hand firmly against the tailbone with fingers wide apart and shake the buttocks to relax the muscles. Then press firmly with all your weight pushing down against the tailbone.

Slide both hands up the back with a series of medium presses along the sides of the spine. Start at the top of the back on the muscles between the shoulder blades and the spine, then work outward on the shoulder muscles. Make several strokes down the neck and across the shoulders, then make small firm circles with the thumbs along the muscles, tracing the muscle structure.

Now place your palms at the top of the back, and work down the back, pressing deeply on the muscles on either side of the spine. Stroke over the hips, and gently up the sides to the armpits, then repeat firmly. Repeat the up-and-down backstrokes several times.

Over the lower back use the thumbs in a kneading motion, then press very firmly with the heel of both hands on the lower end of the spine. Still pushing firmly, work up the spine with steady pressures. Slide down again with the tips of your fingers digging into the two grooves on either side of the spine. Repeat the two-hand push up the spine, this time followed by a light stroke down the back.

Finish using a single light stroke from the head down to the buttocks, then down both legs, then from the back down both arms.

SHOWER MASSAGE—A WARNING

The popular new shower attachments that produce high-intensity pulsating water streams feel great on your back. But, says Dr. Sidney Richman, of Hartford, Connecticut, when directed at the neck area, the stream of water may impinge on special nerve endings and cause a person to faint, or in older persons even trigger a stroke. Warn your family not to direct the massage stream to the neck area.

38 First Aid for the Injured Spine

Improper treatment in the first few minutes after a spinal cord injury can mean death or paralysis for life. And the number of such occurrences is not small—care and rehabilitation of spinal cord injuries is the second most costly medical expense to the American public. How many of the victims could have been saved by proper first-aid care will never be known.

Automobile accidents account for the largest number of spinal cord injuries and deaths. Other causes—diving accidents, football injuries, gunshot wounds, and falls, including those from skateboards.

Whatever the cause of the injury, according to the American College of Emergency Physicians, the period between the accident and the patient's arrival in the emergency department of the hospital is critical—an estimated 25 percent of the fatal complications occur during this time.

Any time there is a violent injury to the head, neck, or spine, whether from a fall, a blow, a collision, or from sudden deceleration, as in an automobile accident, always suspect neck or back damage until proven otherwise.

AT THE SCENE OF AN ACCIDENT

Here are the proper procedures to follow if you suddenly find yourself involved at the scene of an accident with a person who may have a spine injury.

Unless there is danger of fire or an explosion, do not move the victim. Leave him where he is.

Send someone to summon a physician or an ambulance.

Check to see if the victim is breathing. If not, provide mouth-to-mouth resuscitation.

If there is extensive bleeding, apply clean cloths *gently* to stop bleeding.

Cover the injured person to keep him warm and help counteract shock.

Don't do anything else. Do not put a pillow under his head. Do not bend or twist him in any way. Do not try to pull him out of a wrecked car. Don't lift him or move him.

Do not rush him to the hospital. Wait for an ambulance or physician to come to the victim.

If it is necessary to move the victim, do it with great care to avoid any possibility of further damage to the spinal cord. Do not let the head bend forward or tilt sideways. For an emergency stretcher, use a door or wide plank of wood that is rigid. Put it alongside the victim. Have one person kneel and grasp the victim's head firmly between both hands while others grasp the victim's clothing at hips and shoulder, sliding the victim carefully onto the stretcher, moving the entire body and head stiffly with no bending anywhere. Put rolled cloths or sweaters as padding on the sides of the head to prevent rolling. Tie the body to the stretcher in several places. If an ambulance is not available and the victim must be transported, use a truck or station wagon with a flat floor. Drive slowly since bumps or jolts can cause injury.

LATE SIGNS THAT COULD MEAN BRAIN OR SPINE INJURY

Any time a victim has been in a serious accident, even though he has not lost consciousness and shows no signs of injury, he should be taken to the hospital for prompt examination for hidden injuries.

Afterward, even if examination showed no evident damage, the person should be observed closely. Usually delayed evidence of injury will show up in twenty-four hours, but can sometimes appear days later.

Medical help should be obtained immediately if any of the

following signs occur in someone who has had a head or back injury:

inability to move fingers, toes, or other parts of the body

tingling or numb feeling in any part of the body

blood or other fluid coming from mouth, ears, or nose

nausea or vomiting

disturbance in vision, such as double vision, blurring, or difficulty in focusing the eyes

unequal size of pupils of eyes, or pupils that are very dilated or contracted to pinpoints

headache

unusual sleepiness or drowsiness with difficulty in rousing the person

convulsions or blanking-out episodes

difficulty in breathing

speech difficulties

strange behavior or changes in personality or mental ability

HIDDEN FRACTURES

Sometimes it is not the entire backbone that breaks but just a small part of one vertebra. This can happen very easily if a person has bones weakened by a disease such as tuberculosis of the bones or bone infection. Fractures can even occur as the result of violent muscle action in sports or in a convulsion, or from a person falling and landing hard on their feet. Many such fractures go unrecognized at the time of occurrence and are only found later when the patient goes to the doctor with a complaint of persistent pain, or is not able to stand straight.

Here is another type of hidden fracture—a patient goes to the emergency room with a back injury; the doctor finds one spinal fracture, and looks no further. Actually where there's one spinal fracture, there is often likely to be another, says Dr. Joel Rosen, of Northwestern University, and co-director of the Midwest Regional Spinal Cord Injury Care System, in Chicago. There is always the possibility of more than one fracture, he warned physicians in *Emergency Medicine*. He recommended that all patients with spinal cord injuries get X-rays of the entire spine right away. Additional hidden fractures might not generate symptoms at first, he said, but later could turn out to be something very serious.

IN THE EMERGENCY ROOM

Whether the back injury patient is paralyzed for life or can be rehabilitated is not only determined by how he is treated at the scene of the accident but also by how he is treated in the emergency room at the hospital. "Here in the emergency room the ultimate rehabilitation potential of the patient is determined by the avoidance of several mistakes which commonly occur during the period of emergency and acute medical and nursing care," says Dr. Thomas A. Kelley, Jr., of the University of Louisville, Kentucky.

The primary rule in the early care of the patient with spinal cord injuries is to avoid movement of the back, he said, and this rule is commonly broken when a patient is brought to an emergency room, especially when the patient is transferred from a stretcher to an examining table without proper support. Examination can be done, and should be done, while the patient is still on the stretcher, says Dr. Kelley. And the clothing should be cut off while the patient is on the stretcher to avoid movement.

NEWEST TECHNIQUES MAY HELP REVERSE SPINAL CORD INJURY

For the first time in medical history it looks as though something can be done to partially reverse the effects of spinal cord injury. The something: in the first few hours after injury a surgeon cools the area where the spinal cord was injured by slowly filling the wound with ice-cold salt solution. The cooling is done in the operating room to about 20 degrees centigrade for three hours.

When there is an injury, all the damage is not done to the spinal cord at once, according to Dr. Robert White, neurosurgeon at Case Western Reserve University School of Medicine in Cleveland. There is slow tissue breakdown after the injury that eventually destroys the cord. During the time lag, much of the tissue damage can be stopped, he says. The improved recovery that was first shown by Dr. White in animals when he was at the Mayo Clinic has now been shown to produce improvement in nerve function in human patients. But treatment has to be within four to six hours of the injury, he says.

DMSO in spinal injuries. Dr. J. C. de la Torre, associate professor in the department of neurological surgery at the University of Miami School of Medicine, in Florida, reports, "DMSO is a legitimate prescription item in the U.S. for interstitial cystitis. The FDA has approved clinical trials for DMSO in head and spinal cord injuries as well as brain stroke, in university centers located in Oregon, Florida, California, Illinois, and Washington, D.C.

"Our experience with DMSO in spinal cord injuries in animals suggests that complex mechanisms are involved, but stated simply, DMSO may work by keeping open the blood vessels which normally clog within the cord tissues following severe trauma," he says.

"Work in experimental spinal cord injury in animals suggests that DMSO can increase motor recovery following injury, decrease the nerve tissue damage, and even prevent permanent paralysis in treated animals," de la Torre says.

Nerve grafts show promise. At Georgetown University a research team has succeeded in getting dogs to walk again after they have had their spinal cords severed, inducing paralysis. Doctors took nerve segments from the legs of the animals and implanted them in the gaps of the severed cord. Result: Regeneration across the nerve graft; 5 of 40 dogs have been able to walk again.

Spinal cord regeneration in Russia. In 1976 a controversial report was given by neuroanatomist Levon Martinian, of the Orbeli Physiology Institute in the USSR, that a severed spinal cord could be regenerated with injections of enzymes into the cord. The work was first done in laboratory animals, allowing them to move again; then, he said, it was repeated in paraplegics and they were able to walk again.

But since then, Russian researchers say there is only one in 1,000 chances of improvement; only ten patients so far actually have been treated, and no one seems to be sure whether there has really been any improvement. Dr. Veniamin U. Ugriumov, director of the Polenov Neurological Institute in Leningrad, discourages paraplegics from seeking such help at this time.

HALO HELPS AVOID SURGERY IN NECK INJURY

A device that straps around the back and chest and holds the head rigid in a metal halo headband is making it possible for some victims of severe neck injury to avoid what formerly would have been necessary surgery. The halo cast was developed to im-mobilize injured spines before surgical fusion was done; now, says a Mayo Clinic team, the cast has been found to make it possible to *avoid* surgery in many instances. The doctors, Rudolph Klassen, William MacCarty III, and Michael Wood, said the halo cast also resulted in shorter hospital stays and much better healing of bro-ken neck bones. Patients had to wear the halo cast an average of eighty-two days.

DEVICES TO HELP BROKEN BACKS HEAL

A man fell four stories, broke his back, and was immediately paralyzed. When he was brought in to the operating room, Dr. Reuben Hoppenstein, at Beekman-Downtown Hospital in New York, opened the spine and found it was literally in two pieces. Then and there he devised an internal splint made of stainless steel and acrylic cement to bridge over and hold the spine to-gether. Four months later the patient was miraculously walking. Since then, the splint has been used in many patients with broken backs, allowing those who formerly would have been instant paraplegics to walk again. The operation must be done within six hours of the injury, Dr. Hoppenstein says. With the splint, the spine heals so fast the patient can usually sit up in a chair in a matter of days instead of months, he says. The device can also be used for broken necks. One seventeen-year-old boy broke his neck diving into a swimming pool. According to Dr. Hoppenstein, treatment usually would have required tongs in the head, traction on a frame for six weeks, and a rigid cervical collar for two to three months. Instead he left the hospital after only a week.

A similar device made of a stainless-steel rod is sometimes used effectively for broken spines. The rod can range from a few inches to about two feet in length and is clamped to the spine to hold it rigid after surgeons have corrected spinal damage. The patient is often ready for rehabilitation within ten days rather than spending six months motionless in bed or in a cast. The rod may be removed later or left in. In most cases, patients still have enough movement to bend over easily.

A Polish orthopedic surgeon reports he is obtaining good re-sults in spinal fractures using rows of coil springs set up on both sides of the spine. Dr. Marian Weiss, professor and chairman of the department of rehabilitation at the Warsaw School of Medicine, says the stainless-steel springs and hooks are usually left in place for life. Each spring runs from two vertebrae above the fracture to two below and brings about gradual and continuous correction of the fracture. Patients can usually begin rehabilitation training within two weeks after surgery, he says.

NEW FREE FACILITY FOR CHILDREN

The Shriners Hospitals for Crippled Children have just announced a facility to treat children with spinal cord injuries caused by accidents or by tumors. The Spinal Cord Injury Center is at Shriners Hospital for Crippled Children in Philadelphia. It provides free surgical and rehabilitation care for spinal cord injured patients from infancy to age 18.

39 Anatomy of Your Back

The back is really an engineering marvel. It has thirty-one pairs of nerves branching out to all parts of the body and going to and from the brain, thus handling every sensation for pain, touch, heat, and cold, and every signal to your muscles for action. It has three layers of sheathing to protect the nerves, a fluid bath to absorb shock, a bony housing of thirty-three vertebrae which supports most of the body weight, allows us to stand up and still bend, twist and swivel the head to look down at the ground, up at the stars, or over the shoulder.

The spine has an S-shape brilliantly designed to act as its own shock absorber, and for additional shock absorption has disks between each vertebra, something like jelly-filled doughnuts with a tough outer cartilage covering and a jelly-like interior that cushions every step we take. And there are more than 400 intricately connected muscles and 1,000 ligaments supporting the system, giving us shape, support, and most of our ability to move.

Here's how the lineup of your back goes, starting from the top and working down.

The Cervical Spine

The neck region. It has seven vertebrae, the topmost one called the Atlas supports your head, finely balancing it on the top of the spine. The cervical vertebrae mostly make it possible for you to move your head through a wide range of positions. The last cervical vertebra, C7, is where you feel the big bump at the back of your neck between your shoulders.

The Thoracic or Dorsal Spine

This is your midback spine running from the bottom of your neck to your waist. It consists of twelve vertebrae. Primary function—to connect to and support the ribs.

The Lumbar Spine

The lower back region. The five large vertebrae of this region support most of the body weight and work like a five-piece pivot between the upper and lower parts of the body. It absorbs most of the stress and strain of the back and is the area that most frequently gives trouble.

The Sacrum

The five sacral vertebrae are actually fused into one solid triangular structure. It is connected at the top to the last lumbar vertebra and on the sides to the pelvis. The two big bones making up each side of the pelvis are called the ilia. They are connected to the sacrum by ligaments, forming the famous sacroiliac joint. The sacrum and pelvis provide the solid base to the spine for support, provide support for internal abdominal organs such as the bladder, intestines, and uterus, and provide a place for your hipbones to attach your legs to your body. Although the sacroiliac joint has often been blamed for backache, it seldom causes trouble except in some cases of arthritis or if injured.

The Coccyx

Your tailbone. It consists of four vertebrae fused together. It doesn't do much except give some connection to the small rectal muscles that control bowel movements. The tailbone is actually the remnant of what was once a tail in early evolution.

THE DIFFERENCE BETWEEN LIGAMENTS AND TENDONS

Ligaments connect bones to bones.

Tendons connect muscles to bones.

It's ligaments that connect the little projections of the vertebrae together to provide support as you move forward and bend backward and to prevent you from tipping over sideways when you stand up.

WHAT TO KNOW ABOUT YOUR MUSCLES

A muscle tenses and gets shorter when it does its work. It relaxes and gets longer when resting. The really neat design scheme is that muscles always work in pairs—if a muscle contracts to bend your back to the right, then the opposite muscle has to be relaxed to let the back bend. The teamwork can happen automatically because when the nerve impulse sends the signal to make one muscle work, it also sends an inhibitory impulse to the opposing muscle so it will *not* contract.

It's when your muscles are strained with too hard a pull or too long a constant contraction that you can have pain.

The four major muscle groups of the back are as follows:

The spine extensors. These muscles are in layers and are attached to the spine, pelvis, and ribs.

The lateral muscles. These are located along each side of the spine. The two most important are the quadratus lumborum, which balances the sideways motions of the spine, and the psoas major which flexes the trunk and continues down to the hip joint to rotate the hips.

Abdominal muscles. These sheets of muscle support the abdomen and help support and balance the movements of the back.

Hip muscles. These are connected to the pelvis and the spine. They help you flex your hips by raising your thigh, help you balance on your two polelike legs, walk, climb, and run, and help determine your posture.

THE NERVES INSIDE YOUR SPINAL CORD

Your spinal cord is the computer center for your entire nervous system. Nerve roots come and go out of the spinal cord at each segment and serve the parts of the body at that level. The nerves are numbered in relation to the level from which they exit the spine. There are eight cervical (C) nerves, twelve thoracic (T) nerves, five lumbar (L) nerves, and five sacral (S) nerves. The two most significant groups of spinal nerves are C 5 to T 1, which go to the arms and hands, and T 12 to S 4, which go to the legs and feet.

If there is an injury to the spinal cord or damage from a tumor or other pressure on the cord and its nerve roots, a doctor can figure out at exactly what level of the spinal cord the damage has occurred by what areas of the body are paralyzed or otherwise affected.

All the impulses that signal muscles to contract and perform in the body pass through the spinal cord and out the various nerve roots to the body. And all the impulses carrying sensations from the skin go to the spinal cord by way of the nerve roots and up the spinal cord to the centers in the brain that interpret the sensations.

HOW YOUR BACK WAS FORMED AND GREW

The muscles, bones, and nerves of your back started forming and growing when you were a tiny human embryo still in your mother's womb. You started when a sperm and egg joined and formed one single cell. Then this cell divided and made two cells, and these divided and made four and these divided and made eight, then sixteen, then thirty-two—until the tiny speck that was you was a hollow ball of dividing cells. Then, like a crease in a man's hat, the ball folded in upon itself. And where that crease was, the cells started to differentiate. One end of the crease started to swell a bit where your head would be. And a speck appeared where your eye would be, and when you as an embryo were about four weeks old—less than one quarter inch long—a tiny tubelike structure began to beat—your heart. At the same time your muscle cells started to form, and your embryo bone cells began to absorb various minerals that would later make them hard. Also at about the fourth week, small swellings appeared along your sides that would slowly become your arms and legs. And soon little indentations appeared, dividing one pair of buds into future hands and another pair into feet. And this is the time your spine started forming. Your back and other muscles began developing in the early fifth or sixth week. Your spine began to harden at six to eight weeks. By the end of the fourth month, your muscles were able to produce movement.

Amazingly, as your back and other parts of your body developed, you went through the same stages in development that the human race went through in evolutionary history. The earliest embryonic stages of development during our nine months in utero have a definite resemblance to the stages of human evolutionary development over the course of hundreds of thousands of years.

This concept is expressed in a catchy three-word phrase to which every student of embryology is exposed: "Ontogeny recapitulates phylogeny."

"Ontogeny"—the development of the fertilized egg; "recapitulates"—repeats; "phylogeny"—the evolutionary history of the species. Ontogeny recapitulates phylogeny means that in the course of their development, your embryonic structures briefly resembled those same structures of other animals in earlier stages of evolution. The spinal cord, for instance, resembles in its early development the soft, simple spinal cord of the larvalike animal called an Amphioxus, and only later begins to look like a human spinal cord. The developing heart of the human embryo begins as a one-chamber pulsating tube just as it is in lower animals; then it develops into the more complicated heart we know. The spine of the human embryo even has a "tail" which is reabsorbed and disappears before birth.

Childhood and Adolescence

At birth all the muscles and bones of the adult human are present, but they still have a lot of growing to do. The long bones of the arms and legs grow by forming new cartilage where the shaft of the bone meets the head. This cartilage hardens to bone, then new cartilage is formed, gradually making the long bone longer and longer. Then, as adulthood is reached, the long shaft and the rounded head unite and the entire bone is firmly and permanently hardened.

The curve of the spine changes too. In the embryo the spinal column is shaped like a shallow letter C. Then the curve starts to change and continues to change through childhood until it resembles an elongated S in the adolescent. Actually this S-shape appears in stages. The first curve develops in the neck region about the time the infant tries to expand his horizon of vision and holds his head more erect. The second curve in the small of the back starts to form when the child begins to sit up, and develops further when he begins to creep. It is almost completely developed by the time he stands.

HOW OUR SPINES GET SHORTER EVERY DAY

Your spine shortens in two ways. As you get older the disks between the vertebrae get slightly thinner and lose some of their resilience, so your vertebrae are not held quite as far apart. Thus, an older man or woman will be slightly shorter than he or she was in youth. If the spine has also lost some of its bony material, or the person has developed a curve in the back or poor posture, the effect can be intensified to the point that he or she can actually be several inches shorter.

Your spine also shortens every day as you move about because the pressures of body weight and movement compact the jellylike material in the disks, so we are all a trifle shorter in the evening than in the morning. The bounciness of the disks—and our height—are back by morning.

The opposite changes were seen in the backs of astronauts. Scientists were astonished to learn that astronauts, when relieved of the physical stresses on their disks in space, had increased water in the disks to such an extent that they returned to earth two inches taller than when they left!

Glossary of Terms

A

acetabulum—The socket of the pelvic bone.

ACTH—Adrenocorticotropic hormone, a secretion of the pituitary gland which stimulates the adrenal glands to greater activity. This causes an increase of the adrenal cortex hormones, including cortisone.

adductor—Any muscle that pulls a bone toward the midline of the body. The adductor that goes from the pubic bone to the thigh bone is called the adductor longus.

adrenal glands—Endocrine glands that rest on the top of each kidney.

Adrenalin—A trade name for the substance secreted by the adrenal gland. This hormone becomes more plentiful in reactions of fear, rage, flight, or fight. Also called epinephrine.

amyotonia congenita—A disease of muscles, present at birth, and marked by extreme weakness and atrophy. Also called *Oppenheim's disease*.

ankylosing spondylitis—A disease of the spine that has many of the characteristics of rheumatoid arthritis.

anomaly—An anatomical structure that is not normal.

aorta—The large main artery running from the heart down along the front of the backbone.

arthralgia—Pain in the joints without inflammation.

arthritis—Inflammation of a joint.

atlas—The first cervical (neck) vertebra; its major function is to support the skull.

B

benign—Mild and not dangerous. As applied to tumors it means a type that stays local and does not spread.

biceps—A prominent muscle on the front side of the upper arm that extends from the shoulder and wing-bone to the arm bone.

bursae—Small gliding sacs lying between tendons or other moving structures and some fixed part. They lubricate moving areas.

bursitis—An irritation in a bursa. In the earlier stages the bursa becomes tense and swollen. Later calcium may be deposited in the bursa and make its walls thick and gritty (calcified bursitis).

C

cartilage—Gristle; a form of connective tissue that is firm, but not hard and strong like bone. It usually covers the end of a joint and acts as a cushion.

cauda equina—The lower end of the spinal cord as it fans out to form the fifth lumbar, all of the sacral, and the coccygeal nerves. Cauda equina means *horse's tail* in Latin.

cervical ribs—Extra ribs sometimes abnormally present in the neck area.

cervical traction—A pull exerted against the head by means of a special head halter attached to a rope and pulley weight.

coccygeal—Refers to the part of the spine that constitutes the tailbone or coccyx.

coccygodynia—Pain in the region of the tailbone or coccyx.

colchicine—Medicine produced from a plant known as the autumn crocus; used to control acute attacks of gout because of its ability to reduce inflammation.

congenital—Condition present from the time of birth.

corticosteroids—Powerful anti-inflammatory drugs used for short periods to reduce inflammation of the joints. These drugs are produced from a substance found in the outer layer of the adrenal glands, located just above the kidneys.

cyclophosphamide—An immunosuppressive drug, similar to those used in organ transplant operations, used with caution and only in carefully selected arthritic patients; not yet recommended for general use.

D

discogram—X-ray made with injection by needle of opaque material into the disk between two vertebrae.

E

endocrines—Chemicals secreted internally which have great influence on the growth and physiology of the body. They are secreted directly into the blood stream.

endocrinologist—Physician who specializes in the diagnosis and treatment of illnesses related to the glands of internal secretion.

epinephrine—Adrenalin.

erector spinae muscles—The large muscles which run along the full length of the back of the spine. These are the strongest of the back muscles and the most important for holding the back erect.

extension—Arching the trunk or neck backward, or moving a joint to make the angle formed by its parts approach a straight line.

F

flat feet—Feet whose supporting muscles have grown too weak to do their job and have allowed the normal arches of the feet to settle. Also called *pes planus*.

flexion—Bending the trunk or neck forward, or moving a joint to make the angle formed by its parts smaller.

flexor muscle—Muscle that bends a joint.

frozen shoulder—A stiffening of the shoulder joint due to inflammation or immobility of the arm.

G

gastroc-soleus—Refers to two muscles: the gastrocnemius, the large calf muscle that goes from the back of the thigh bone to the heel bone, and the soleus, located just in front of it.

gluteus maximus—The large fleshy muscle at the back of the hip that extends from the outer part of the thigh bone to the hipbone.

gold treatment—The use of gold salts to relieve or reduce the symptoms of arthritis.

gout—A disease that affects the joints and kidneys, caused by abnormal body chemistries that produce an excess amount of uric acid.

H

hamstring muscle—Large muscles at the back of the thigh attaching to the hip above and leg below.

Heberden's nodes—Bony enlargements of the end joints of the fingers.

hypertrophic arthritis—Ridging and spurring of bone near joints as evidence of wear and tear of these areas.

I

idiopathic—Without a known cause.

iliopsoas—A composite of two muscles, the psoas major and the iliacus. The psoas major goes from the backbone to the thigh bone. The iliacus is a flat triangular muscle which extends from the hipbone to the thigh bone.

indomethacin—An anti-inflammatory drug.

insomnia—The inability to sleep.

intervertebral disk—The spongy fibrous cushions that join adjacent vertebral bodies and give spring to the spine.

J

joints—Connections fastening bones together.

K

Klippel-Feil's syndrome—Congenital fusion of some or all of the neck vertebrae into one mass.

Kümmell's disease—Progressive wedging of the body of a vertebra after injury. This disease usually represents an unrecognized or untreated fracture.

kyphosis—Deformity of the back in which there is a backward arching of the spine. This is most common in the upper back.

L

lesion—Tissue or part of an organ damaged by injury or disease, usually with partial loss of function, for example, a bruise or broken bone.

ligaments—Sheets and strands of dense fibers that keep the joint ends together, completely enclosing the joint in a capsule-like arrangement.

lordosis—Backward curvature of the lumbar spine.

lumbago—The old-fashioned term for pain in the lower part of the back.

lumbar—Lower portion of the spine attaching to the pelvis.

lumbosacral joint—The connection between the last lumbar and the first sacral vertebra.

M

malignant—The type of tumor which tends to spread throughout the body.

masseur—A man who practices massage.

masseuse—A woman who practices massage.

meninges—The three layers of tissue that cover the brain and spinal cord.

meningitis—Inflammation of the covering of the brain and spinal cord.

menisci—Fibrocartilages found in the knee and some other joints.

metatarsal bar—A leather strip across the front of the shoe behind the ball of the foot, designed to place more weight on the arch of the foot and less on the toes.

methyl methacrylate—A cement used to form a synthetic bone base to connect the hip or knee bones of patients with metal and plastic joints.

mixed arthritis—When rheumatoid arthritis and osteoarthritis occur at the same time. This is usually caused by rheumatoid arthritis, which can lead to secondary osteoarthritis due to injury to the joints.

morphine—A narcotic drug obtained from opium and used for the relief of severe pain. If used for a prolonged period, it produces a strong addiction.

myalgia—Pain in the muscles.

myelogram—X-ray with injection by needle of opaque material into the space that contains the spinal cord or nerve roots.

N

neural arch—The bony ring extending back from each vertebra, surrounding and protecting part of the spinal cord or the spinal nerves.

neuralgia—Severe pain along the course of a nerve not associated with any obvious or demonstrable structural changes in the nerve.

neuritis—Inflammation of a nerve.

neuroma—A benign tumor of a nerve.

nucleus pulposus—The semiliquid gelatinous center of an intervertebral disk. Its major function is to provide a cushion between the vertebrae. At times it ruptures out to press against nerve roots and cause back or leg pain.

O

osteoarthritis—A disease of the joints that involves a breakdown of cartilage and other tissues that make it possible for a joint to move normally. Inflammation may or may not be present.

osteopetrosis—An inherited disease characterized by a generalized increase in bone density that begins during growth. There are at least two different forms, one of early onset with poor prognosis, the other of late onset, little disability, and normal life expectancy.

P

pelvis—The large bones in the middle of the body supporting the trunk and supported by the femurs (thigh bones) at the hips.

phenylbutazone—A drug used to treat acute outbreaks of arthritic pain for a short period of time.

physiatrist—A physician who specializes in physical medicine; often develops a program of exercises for arthritic or other back patients to help prevent crippling.

physical therapist—A person trained to treat patients by physical means, such as heat, massage, exercise, whirlpool baths, ultraviolet light, etc.

pigeon breast—A congenital deformity of the breastbone characterized by a bulging of its center.

pilonidal cyst—A walled-off pocket of dimpled-in skin over the sacrum. These tend to grow hair inside and become infected in adults to form abscesses or sinuses; can be treated by surgery.

polo belt—A broad-backed belt gripping the pelvis, designed to protect and support the low back area.

posteriolateral sclerosis—A disease of the spinal cord that causes numbness and weakness of the arms and legs.

prednisone—A powerful corticosteroid sometimes used in the treatment of arthritis. It must be used under a doctor's direction to prevent serious side effects.

primary osteoarthritis—Osteoarthritis that occurs without having been influenced by any known event or injury; starts by itself.

procaine—The same as Novocain, a local anesthetic.

pronate—To turn inward.

psoriatic arthritis—A disease in which psoriasis is complicated by arthritis that has the characteristics of rheumatoid arthritis.

pyknodysostosis—Disease that afflicted the painter Toulouse-Lautrec. The stature is short, primarily because of short extremities. There is increased liability to fracture.

Q

quadratus lumborum—The four-sided muscle that forms a flat sheet on each side of the spinal column and goes from the lower border of the last rib to the crest of the hipbone.

quadriceps—Muscle composed of the rectus femoris, the vastus lateralis, and the vastus medialis. They go down the thigh from the hip joint to the kneecap.

R

referred pain—Pain felt some distance away from its cause. For example, pain in the knees caused by an osteoarthritic hip.

Reiter's syndrome—A disease involving inflammation of the urethra, eyelids, and arthritis in several joints.

remission—State when a disease appears to have gone away by itself, usually temporarily.

resting splints—Splints designed to be used when the patient is resting or sleeping.

rheumatic fever—A disease caused by streptococcus infection that results in inflammation of the joints and may cause damage to the heart.

rheumatism—Unspecific or unexplained aches and pains that may occur in joints or muscles or both; often used to mean arthritis.

rheumatoid arthritis—Inflammation of the joints in which the whole body can be affected. Symptoms include stiffness and aching of joints, general fatigue, and loss of appetite.

rheumatologist—A physician who specializes in the treatment and management of patients with arthritis.

S

sacroiliac—The joints or articulations between the sacrum and the two ilia of the pelvis, bound together by ligaments.

sacrum—The wedge-shaped bone at the back of the pelvis supporting the lumbar spine and ending in the coccyx (tailbone).

sciatica—Pain along the sciatic nerve or part of it; may be in the buttocks, leg, or toes.

scoliosis—A side-to-side or lateral curvature of the spine.

secondary osteoarthritis—Osteoarthritis that occurs because of wear and tear or injury to one or more joints.

slipped disk—A bulging of part of the cushion disk between the vertebrae. Also called a ruptured disk, a protruded disk, or herniated nucleus pulposus.

spina bifida—A congenital failure of the bone covering the spinal cord to form completely.

spinal cord—The main trunk line for nerve messages to and from the brain. It extends from the skull down into the lumbar area of the spine, protected by the vertebrae.

spinal nerves—Nerves running from the spinal cord to various parts of the body. There are thirty-one pairs of spinal nerves. (There are also twelve pairs of cranial nerves running directly from the brain to the head and other parts of the body.)

spinal rachischisis—A congenital defect in which the back is open, exposing the spinal cord.

spine fusion—An operation in which bone grafts are placed in the back to render two or more of its segments permanently rigid.

splint—A rigid structure applied to a part of the body to immobilize that area.

spondylolisthesis—An unhealed fracture across the back of a vertebra, usually the last lumbar, which makes this part of

the back unstable. It is usually congenital but may be caused
by an injury.

sprain—A wrenching of a joint which tears or severely stretches
the ligaments with bleeding and swelling.

Sprengel's deformity—Congenital elevation of a shoulder blade.

strain—Overuse or mild stretching of a part of the body.

striated muscles—The voluntary muscles of the body.

supraspinatus muscle—A muscle in the shoulder that pulls the
arm overhead.

T

tendinitis—Inflammation of a tendon.

torticollis—A deformity in which the neck is tilted to the side and
twisted; also called wryneck.

transverse process of a vertebra—Bony projection to the vertebra
for muscle attachments.

trauma—An injury.

U

uric acid—A chemical compound in the form of salts that is
found in the joints of gout sufferers. It is also the major con-
stituent of kidney stones.

V

vertebrae—The bones of the spine.

vitalium—An alloy composed of cobalt, chromium, and molyb-
denum, used in the manufacture of artificial joints.

Directory of Free and Nearly Free Health Information and Services Relating to the Back

A GUIDE OF WHERE TO GO FOR INFORMATION AND FURTHER HELP ON YOUR SPECIFIC BACK PROBLEMS

There are hundreds of services available in this country, free or almost free, that the public, and often even the medical profession, is not completely aware of. Voluntary health organizations, medical schools, hospitals, and government agencies are available to help you with almost any problem.

You can write to them for booklets, write or call them about specific problems, and often can use their diagnostic and treatment facilities for a nominal fee or sometimes for nothing. Many also give financial help to patients.

Check your own area for services and information at hospitals, medical schools, agencies, and neighborhood clinics near you, city and state health departments, and local branches of the U.S. Public Health Service.

We have listed the addresses of the national offices of organizations in this directory. But many agencies also have local chapters, so check your telephone directory to see if there is a chapter in your city where you can visit personally to discuss your problem. If you cannot find a local chapter in your area, write to the national headquarters and ask them for help.

To find government services, you usually should look under the name of the city or state. For example, if you live in Chicago, you would look under several listings: *Chicago, City of; Cook, County of; Illinois, State of;* and *United States.* Under these you will then find Department of Health, etc.

If you are writing for a booklet, you will get faster service if you enclose a stamped, self-addressed business-sized envelope.

AGING

Administration of Aging
    U.S. Department of Health, Education and Welfare
    Washington, D.C. 20201
National Geriatrics Society
    165 North Pearl Street
    Albany, New York 12207
American Association of Retired Persons
    1090 K Street, N.W.
    Washington, D.C. 20049
        Information on aging, pharmacy, nursing-home services, and health, life, and auto insurance programs.
American Geriatrics Society
    10 Columbus Circle
    New York, New York 10019
Gerontological Society
    110 South Central Avenue
    Clayton, Missouri 63105
National Council of Senior Citizens
    1627 K Street, N.W.
    Washington, D.C. 20006
        Sponsors Medicare supplemental insurance and drug-discount programs for members. Low-cost travel benefits.
National Council on the Aging
    1828 L Street, N.W.
    Washington, D.C. 20036
        Extensive library of literature on aging. A national directory of housing for older people. $5.50.

ARTHRITIS

The Arthritis Foundation
    3400 Peachtree Street, N.E.
    Atlanta, Georgia 30326

Clinic, home-care programs, and centers for care and rehabilitation to arthritis patients. Many chapters also have facilities for occupational therapy. Information on rheumatic conditions.

National Institute of Arthritis and Metabolic Diseases
    Office of Information
    Bethesda, Maryland 20014
        Information on causes, prevention, and treatment of various arthritic, rheumatic, collagen, and metabolic diseases.

CHILDREN

American Academy of Pediatrics
    1801 Hinman Avenue
    Evanston, Illinois 60204
American Association for Maternal and Child Health
    116 South Michigan Avenue
    Chicago, Illinois 60603
American School Health Association
    515 East Main Street
    Kent, Ohio 44240
Office of Child Development
    Department of Health, Education and Welfare
    P.O. Box 1182
    Washington, D.C. 20013
National Institute of Child Health and Human Development
    National Institutes of Health
    Bethesda, Maryland 20014
National Association of Children's Hospitals and Related Institutions
    1308 Delaware Avenue
    Wilmington, Delaware 19805

FINANCIAL AID

To apply for public assistance, you must appear in person at the Welfare Department center nearest your home. The criteria for receiving public assistance is not enough money to meet the needs of a family, as calculated on a public assistance budget, which is very low. Categories of welfare are:

Home Relief, for a person who does not earn enough money to maintain his family or himself and is unable to secure additional support.

Old Age Assistance, for persons over sixty-five unable to support themselves.

Aid to the Disabled, for persons permanently or totally disabled and unable to support themselves.

Veteran Assistance, for aid to veterans falling under any of the above categories.

Aid to Dependent Children, for children under sixteen, eighteen, or twenty-one if in school, whose parents cannot support them. Aid is also given to the mother.

FOOT CARE

American Podiatry Association
20 Chevy Chase Circle, N.W.
Washington, D.C. 20015
    Foot-health screening examinations in schools and community health programs. Free literature.

GENETIC COUNSELING

National Genetics Foundation
250 West 57th Street
New York, New York 10019
    Genetic counseling and treatment centers to help people who have, or suspect they have, hereditary diseases. Diagnosis and treatment in family planning.

National Foundation—March of Dimes
P.O. Box 2000
· White Plains, New York 10602
    Genetic counseling and diagnosis. Complete international list of genetic counseling services by area.

HOMEMAKER SERVICES

National Committee on Homemaker Service
12 South Lake Avenue
Albany, New York 12203

Homemaker service programs and advisers to programs.
National Council for Homemaker—Home Health Aide Services
1740 Broadway
New York, New York 10019
Gives care and help to people in their homes.

MEDICAID

Medical Services Administration
Social and Rehabilitation Service
U.S. Department of Health, Education and Welfare
Washington, D.C. 20201
Information on federal and state medical assistance programs.

MEDICINES

Food and Drug Administration
Consumer Enquiry
5600 Fishers Lane
Rockville, Maryland 20852
Information on drug side effects and medicines.
Pharmaceutical Manufacturers Association
1155 15th Street, N.W.
Washington, D.C. 20005
Information on prescription medicines.
Proprietary Association
1700 Pennsylvania Avenue, N.W.
Washington, D.C. 20006
Information on nonprescription medicines.

NURSING HOMES

American Health Care Association
1025 Connecticut Avenue, N.W.
Washington, D.C. 20036
Information on proprietary and nonproprietary nursing homes.
American Association of Homes for the Aging
529 Fourteenth Street, N.W.
Washington, D.C. 20004

NUTRITION THERAPY

Huxley Institute for Biosocial Research
    1114 First Avenue
    New York, New York 10021
International Academy of Metabology
    2236 Suree Ellen Lane
    Altadena, California 91001
International College of Applied Nutrition
    Box 386
    La Habra, California 90631
Academy of Orthomolecular Psychiatry
    1691 Northern Boulevard
    Manhasset, New York 11030
International Academy of Preventive Medicine
    871 Frostwood Drive
    Houston, Texas 77024

OSTEOGENESIS IMPERFECTA

Osteogenesis Imperfecta Foundation
    1231 May Court
    Burlington, North Carolina 27215

OSTEOPATHIC MEDICINE

American Osteopathic Association
    212 East Ohio Street
    Chicago, Illinois 60611

PHYSICAL FITNESS

President's Council on Physical Fitness and Sports
    7th and D Streets, S.W.
    Washington, D.C. 20202
        Promotes home and school exercise programs.

POLIOMYELITIS

Georgia Warm Springs Foundation
    120 Broadway

New York, New York 10005
> Aids sufferers from after-effects of polio.

The National Foundation—March of Dimes
P.O. Box 2000
White Plains, New York 10602
> (Formerly the National Foundation for Infantile Paralysis.) Provides information and aids patients.

REHABILITATION

American Academy of Physical Medicine and Rehabilitation
30 North Michigan Avenue
Chicago, Illinois 60602

American Occupational Therapy Association
251 Park Avenue South
New York, New York 10010

American Physical Therapy Association
1740 Broadway
New York, New York 10019

American Rehabilitation Committee
28 East 21st Street
New York, New York 10010
> Maintains a rehabilitation center for the disabled.

National Information Center for the Handicapped
Box 1492
Washington, D.C. 20013

Association for the Aid of Crippled Children
345 East 46th Street
New York, New York 10017

Association for the Aid of Crippled Children and Adults
239 Park Avenue South
New York, New York 10010

Children's Bureau
Office of Child Development
330 Independence Avenue, S.W.
Washington, D.C. 20201
> Will tell you where there is a clinic in your area that offers services for handicapped children.

Department of Defense
Washington, D.C. 20301

Employs disabled civilians and rehabilitates disabled serv-
icemen and women.
Disabled American Veterans
  1425 East McMillan Street
  Cincinnati, Ohio 45206
    Aids disabled veterans with hospitals, insurance, and
    employment.
Goodwill Industries of America
  1913 N Street, N.W.
  Washington, D.C. 20006
    Provides employment opportunities for the handicapped
    and disabled.
Institute for the Crippled and Disabled
  400 First Avenue
  New York, New York 10010
    Vocational advice for rehabilitation.
Institute of Physical Medicine and Rehabilitation
  400 East 34th Street
  New York, New York 10016
    Homemakers program for disabled.
Paralyzed Veterans of America
  7315 Wisconsin Avenue
  Washington, D.C. 20014
    Many publications including Wheelchair House Plans (50
    cents) and guidebooks for handicapped travelers.
President's Committee on Employment of the Handicapped
  Washington, D.C. 20210
    Promotional opportunities for training and employment
    for the handicapped.
National Association of the Physically Handicapped
  76 Elm Street
  London, Ohio 43140
National Association of Sheltered Workshops and Homebound
  Programs
  1522 K Street
  Washington, D.C. 20005
National Center for Law and the Handicapped
  1235 North Eddy Street
  South Bend, Indiana 46617
    Legal assistance on rights of handicapped persons.

National Easter Seal Society for Crippled Children and Adults
2023 West Ogden Avenue
Chicago, Illinois 60612
>Vocational and educational services. Sheltered workshops, treatment centers, mobile therapy units, camps. "New York City Guide for the Handicapped" lists where to find wheelchair ramps and other special facilities free.

National Rehabilitation Association
1029 Vermont Avenue, N.W.
Washington, D.C. 20005
>Rehabilitation services for the mentally and physically handicapped.

Office of Vocational Rehabilitation
Washington, D.C. 20201
>Information on federal-state programs for rehabilitating handicapped persons.

Shriner's Hospital for Crippled Children
323 North Michigan Avenue
Chicago, Illinois 60601

Shut-In Society, Inc.
11 West 42nd Street
New York, New York 10036
>Provides correspondence and other services for the handicapped.

Sister Kenny Rehabilitation Institute
1800 Chicago Avenue
Minneapolis, Minnesota 55404

U.S. Department of Health, Education and Welfare
Social and Rehabilitation Service
330 C Street, S.W.
Washington, D.C. 20201
>Coordinates government services to the handicapped.

VETERANS' HEALTH CARE

Veterans Administration
810 Vermont Avenue, N.W.
Washington, D.C. 20420
>Benefits for medical treatment to all eligible veterans and certain dependents.

MISCELLANEOUS

American Medical Association
   535 North Dearborn Street
   Chicago, Illinois 60610
      Films, booklets, and other educational information.
American National Red Cross
   Washington, D.C. 20005
      Disaster aid. Local chapters provide services such as driv-
      ing patients to and from treatments.
National Institutes of Health Clinical Center
   Bethesda, Maryland 20014
      A free medical research center for certain chronic condi-
      tions. A physician must recommend the patient and sup-
      ply medical information. Among conditions treated:
      juvenile rheumatoid arthritis, severe obesity, calcium dis-
      orders, abnormal patterns of growth, muscular dystrophy,
      and parkinsonism.
Salvation Army
   120 West 14th Street
   New York, New York 10011
      Residential center for homeless, camping for children,
      senior citizens, and physically handicapped persons.
Superintendent of Documents
   Government Printing Office
   Washington, D.C. 20402
      Clearinghouse for U.S. Government publications on many
      subjects.
Volunteers of America
   340 West 85th Street
   New York, New York 10024
      Aid to the handicapped, clubs and homes for the aged,
      and services for the destitute.

RELIGIOUS ORGANIZATIONS WITH NATIONAL HEALTH AND SOCIAL SERVICES

American Baptist Homes & Hospitals Association
   Valley Forge, Pennsylvania 19481

Catholic Charities
    122 East 22nd Street
    New York, New York 10010
Council of Jewish Federations and Welfare Funds
    315 Park Avenue South
    New York, New York 10010
Federation of Protestant Welfare Agencies
    281 Park Avenue South
    New York, New York 10010
The Lutheran Church–Special Ministries
    315 Park Avenue South
    New York, New York 10010
National Association of Methodist Hospitals & Homes
    1200 Davis Street
    Evanston, Illinois 60201
National Jewish Welfare Board
    145 East 32nd Street
    New York, New York 10022
U.S. Catholic Conference–Bureau of Health and Hospitals
    1312 Massachusetts Avenue, N.W.
    Washington, D.C. 20005

Index